Health is Wealth with Ayurveda

By Susan Holman

Health is Wealth with Ayurveda

A Practical Guide to Restore, Repair and Rejuvenate Your Health

Copyright 2024 © Susan Holman

Published by Susan Coach LLC

www.wellnesschique.com

All rights reserved. No portion of this book may be reproduced in any form without permission from the publisher except as permitted by copyright law. For permission contact susan@susan.coach

ISBN: 978-1-7364437-2-9

Dedication

I dedicate this book to my brother Bob who inspires me every day why this work is so important from his heavenly abode.. I also dedicate this book to the Ayurvedic physicians who have helped me along this incredible journey, including Dr. Kaushik.

DISCLAIMER

This book is not intended to treat, diagnose or prescribe. The information herein is not a substitute for seeing your health care professional. Please consult with your physician or healthcare specialist regarding the suggestions and recommendations made in this book. The use of this book implies your acceptance of this disclaimer.

The publisher and the author make no guarantees covering the level of success you may experience by following the advice and strategies contained in this book and you accept the risk that results will differ for each individual

TABLE OF CONTENTS

INTRODUCTION 1

CHAPTER 1 : Take Back Your Health with Ayurveda 5

CHAPTER 2 : Realize the Value of Your Health 17

CHAPTER 3 : Get to Know Ayurveda 29

CHAPTER 4 : Know Thy Constitution or Dosha 37

CHAPTER 5 : Exercise for Your Dosha 51

CHAPTER 6 : Breathing Exercises / Pranayama 63

CHAPTER 7 : Know Your Kitchen (Herbs, Spices and Plants) 77

CHAPTER 8 : Foods that Boost Digestion 89

CHAPTER 9 : Yoga Nidra / The Five Sheaths 103

CHAPTER 10 : Energy Points and Marma Massage 113

CHAPTER 11 : Let Excellent Health Be Your Guide 125

CHAPTER 12 : Create Community with Your Ayurveda Knowledge 135

REFERENCES 145

GLOSSARY OF AYURVEDIC TERMS 146

ABOUT THE AUTHOR 157

INTRODUCTION

At the time of writing this book and for many decades now, we have seen a decline in the health of people in the United States. The upsurge in pre-diabetes, diabetes, obesity and cancer rates is out of control. In most cases, it is downright preventable if people were educated as to how these diseases arise from lifestyle and the foods we eat. It seems to mostly come from poor diet and nutritional habits layered on with a tendency to overmedicate. We live in a country where pharmaceutical companies can pitch directly to the consumer in advertising. This has a hypnotic effect on people, making them dependent on a drug to solve just about any medical issue. There is a time and a place for medication, but before a doctor recommends medication, they should be asking questions about the person's health to see if natural remedies can help to boost the immune system. If so, then medical professionals will need to scale way back on the prescribing of meds and move toward health education. Health care professionals can benefit from the knowledge of herbs and nutrition that derive from Ayurveda. Then they can boost their clients' immune systems naturally.

My own primary care physician in NYC gives lectures to other MDs about how they should be taught how to prescribe healthy meals to patients. He also suggests that hospitals start having gardens in which to harvest fresh foods in order to teach by example for their patients. He talked about the lack of quality in hospital food that is not healing the patient. The times are changing in some circles slowly but surely.

I have witnessed firsthand in my own family how poor dietary habits have led to compromised immune systems with the people I care about. I saw my brother's health deteriorate from poor habits that could have been reversed through proper access to the tools and knowledge of natural healing that Ayurveda offers.

I have also lost relatives who were prescribed medications that ended up creating other more serious conditions in their bodies. It was disheartening at a young age for me not to be able to help them. It was already too late. If learning by experience is a blessing, then there is hope to correct some of the health problems we are witnessing in our homes and in our cities as well.

The time is ripe for introducing the knowledge of Ayurveda into our health education and wellness systems worldwide. With Ayurveda we have access to ancient natural healing methods that come from some of the earliest known texts of the Vedas on surgery and medicine. The recommendations start from the root of an individual's health by looking at their unique characteristics according to their dosha or bioenergetic and personality traits. Through a series of health questions and pulse reading, natural herbs, spices, plants and foods can be recommended to boost the individual's health to help heal their weak areas.

Ayurvedic recommendations treat the whole person so that their lifestyle is conducive to optimum health. An Ayurvedic expert will help you discover the best times of day to eat for your constitution and what types of food will best serve you. This will all be in the context of what you have going on with your health right now. Recommendations cover a wide variety of lifestyle changes, including exercise modifications, sleep recommendations, self-care and gentle detox methods. These are all complementary to what your primary care physician is doing and will only help to straighten and boost your immune system and overall health.

The climate is ripe for change in the U.S. with metabolic syndromes and neurological disorders on the rise. It is estimated that roughly 35% of the U.S. population has metabolic syndrome. That means that about 1 in 3 people will have a metabolic syndrome of one type. There are risk factors associated with metabolic syndrome which include high blood sugar, high blood pressure, high cholesterol and excessive abdominal fat. This is so incredibly high but it can be comforting to know that there are herbal remedies and dietary recommendations that are powerful yet gentle on the system that can help an individual to overcome these risk factors.

Recent CDC data from 2017-18 also shows that 42.4 % of American adults are obese, which is defined by having a body index of 30% or higher. This is a significant climb from the previous two decades and is only on the rise. Twenty-eight percent of American adults according to a 2018 study have dyslipidemia, which is a key risk factor for cardiovascular disease. Ninety to ninety-five percent of the 34.2 million Americans who have diabetes have Type 2 diabetes according to a 2018 CDC study. There is so much room for improvement in the great American diet, which tends to be high in processed foods and cholesterol. Let's start mapping out a plan with Ayurveda.

Throughout my consultations with clients over the past eight years I have seen that time and money are also contributing factors to their health breakdowns. Lifestyles tend to be overly hectic without the proper organization in a person's day for regeneration of their health. I have direct experience in being treated with Ayurvedic remedies and dietary changes for my own digestive health. I can say that I was able to rid my own body of inflammatory markers that were showing up in my blood after getting vaccinated. It took two months to change my blood back to healthy levels for cholesterol and enzymes through the help of an Ayurvedic physician. This really works and I knew this from the time I started my training as an Ayurvedic consultant back in 2017.

I have always believed in natural healing and medicine but was truly impressed with the vast amounts of plant and herbal classifications that Ayurvedic medicine has. There are many thousands of plant, herb, oil, seed and grain options that can easily encompass a lifetime of learning. I look forward to sharing this information with you as the study of Ayurveda is filled with such promise for fostering good health for many generations to come.

CHAPTER 1

Take Back Your Health with Ayurveda

Life comes at you fast; don't let death do the same thing. The media sells disempowerment for your health, so be careful not to buy it. Prescription drug ads are seductively crafted with great music and acting. It's only at the end of the ad that you hear a disclaimer in a whisper-like tone that the drug may cause seizures, sudden death or thoughts of suicide.

Where have we gone wrong? Who is writing this script? Not you. But one thing is for sure, you are running scared. You have this friend or that friend who has experienced health problems or has lost their battle to some disease. You are googling the symptoms that you hear other people talk about and the result has you reaching for anything outside of yourself to help heal it.

Meet Melody, a busy NYC schoolteacher in her mid-30s who is already considered obese by body mass index standards. To top it off, she also has swollen feet and ankles. She's had some residual post-pandemic habits that fueled her fatigue and eating habits. Her busy life as a teacher has taken her cortisol levels higher and is increasing her stress. She also has feelings of loneliness even though she works with people every day. This is fueling a health decline for Melody that may be unnoticeable at first, but that will have a snowball effect on her health as she continues to live this type of lifestyle. The weight becomes increasingly harder to get off, and the comfort eating is happening so unconsciously that it is creating a false sense of balance for her. Since eating during sugar lows helps to balance hormone and neurotransmitter levels, this is part of her "false sense of balance" and it will escalate into bigger problems down the line.

She starts to take pills to manage her cholesterol and her blood sugar goes up. She thinks they may be connected but still resorted to more prescription pills to alleviate the problem and ends up gaining more weight. Now she becomes depressed and seeks out help for that. Suddenly her health got complicated. They should have a status update on social media for health called "it's complicated" because her health issues just became a whole lot more involved. She is not happy and is starting to ask herself how she could have let her health go. She was smart. She was successful but she was not aware of what she didn't know that could have helped her.

When I started coaching Melody in Ayurveda, her life took a big turn. She was no longer dependent on sources outside of herself to restore her health, she was creating it! Every day she started noticing improvements in her energy, the pounds started to come off and she felt great. When you learn these principles that I call "Ayurveda basics," your life will improve too. You will notice more clarity, energy and overall wellbeing by partaking in the knowledge of Ayurveda. You will benefit greatly from an Ayurvedic consultation which determines your basic constitution. There are three constitutions, *pitta* (fire), *kapha*, (earth) and *vata* (air), and there are combinations of these three to make seven constitutions in total.

In popular Ayurvedic teachings, many people refer to the constitutions as *dosha*. Are you a *pitta, kapha* or *vata dosha*? I would like to clarify that in Sanskrit the word *dosha* literally means "something that can go out of balance or create a problem." So, dosha technically has two contextual meanings. One context describes your general personality traits and bioenergetics, which is the context that I am using throughout this book. The other context in which the 3 types of doshas are being used is to describe a problem in the body where the terms *pitta, kapha* and *vata* are used differently in order to describe a disorder in a body organ or body system. The latter is used in diagnostic contexts and as they come up, I will point them out.

When I became an Ayurvedic consultant, I knew this knowledge would benefit people of all ages with various health conditions and that they would feel empowered about their health. I love educating clients about the incredible health benefits of this wonderful ancient healing method. In India, Ayurveda is recognized as medical knowledge since the roots of the system run very deep. In the U.S., it is recognized as a natural healthcare system but not as medicine, since it has not been established as a form of medical training in the U.S. We do not know a lot about the scope of Ayurveda, which includes an elaborate classification of herbs, spices and essential oils along with Vedic knowledge of human physiology and energy systems. It contains within it an infinite resource of knowledge that can help you restore, rejuvenate and regenerate your health.

Have you ever found yourself questioning your health and longevity? Have you ever wondered if there could be a peaceful, balanced solution to all the "noise" out there in cyberspace about which methods work best to restore your energy naturally? Every day we hear about someone passing away in their prime by heart disease, diabetes, various forms of cancers or a host of immune diseases. Do we have to sit back and take it? Do you find yourself confused by all the natural solutions out there? What if the organic and natural foods in your local stores were simply carbohydrates and sugars in disguise that do nothing to nourish and balance your body? How can you shop smarter? Are you exercising and feeling tired or is it that something is still not right? Maybe you need exercises that are tailored toward not only restoring your strength and flexibility but also your body's energy systems. And, when you delve into the knowledge of Ayurvedic wisdom, you will discover subtle energy systems within that you never knew existed!

In this book I will share with you how applying Ayurvedic techniques to your everyday life will help you feel healthier and more energized and will totally rock your world! You will be amazed at how a centuries-old method of health care is transforming the health and wellness of people who partake. They are feeling more connected to their inner health and how it relates to their outside world than ever before. They enjoy learning about the subtle energy systems of the body and how that influences their digestion, absorption of nutrients, and even the exercises they do! They are treating themselves (clinically and recreationally) to the joys of using essential oils, exotic herbs and healing spices, and natural skincare with things you can find in your fridge.

Today degenerative disease is still on the rise and is particularly high in the United States. The Centers for Disease Control and Prevention, in their data from 2017-2020, suggest that obesity levels in the United States have climbed to 41.9%, with higher prevalence among some socially and economically disadvantaged groups. Everyone knows that obesity contributes to increased risk for type 2 diabetes, degenerative joint disease, sleep problems and hypertension, to name just a few. Your risk for heart disease goes up and you have a host of related problems including swollen legs and feet, lethargy, inflammation and a downcast outlook on life.

In the U.S., with all our wealth, we are quite poor when it comes to our health. There is great potential for changing this when people know what to do. Keeping them in the dark about real health knowledge only exacerbates the problem. In our educational system we haven't learned how to live healthier lives by eating nourishing foods and absorbing these nutrients. So, let's start embracing the idea that you can transform your health and feel more peace of mind in the process. Stop giving your power away to an ad for the next quick fix or something outside of yourself when you can have the answers within yourself. You do have the power.

We all know plenty of people who never felt they had the power to change their health. Take my brother Bob, for example, may he rest in peace. It all started when he was 45 years old. He was on a crash course with his health: smoking 2 packs of hand-rolled cigarettes a day, drinking 10 cups of coffee and eating fatty, cholesterol-rich foods like they were going out of style. He was not obese, but he was setting the stage for heart failure in a big-time way. His diet was empty of nutrients and high in fats and sugars. Eventually he had one heart attack and then a few years later he had a massive heart attack that left him at the crossroads of life. I will never forget this moment. Doctors at Brigham and Women's in Boston gave him two choices: ace a stress test and live on 20+ pills a day or... have a heart transplant! He sounded depressed and wasn't even sure if he wanted to keep living when my sister and I spoke to him on the phone.

My sister decided to bring his two little kids to see him in the hospital (he was going through a divorce), and this ended up being the motivation he needed to keep on going. They saw their daddy hooked up to electrodes and wondered what they were there for as they tried to hug him. Their innocence sparked something in him to ace the stress test. He did ace the test and ended up living on the 20+ pills a day, bypassing the need for a heart transplant! It was abundantly clear that he had to watch his diet and quit smoking. According to his doctors, he had the heart of a degenerating 90-year-old man as he was only living off one artery. He tried quitting smoking and watching his diet for a few months, but eventually old habits started to kick back in. He started sneaking back in the fatty foods and even rolling his own cigarettes. My sister and I jokingly said that he was going to outlive us all as he seemed to be made of cast iron. This was crazy, but fate had something different in store for Bob.

One day he met a new woman and fell in love. Boy, did he ever wish he had taken care of his health! And did I ever wish I could have helped him. My brother had unfortunately tempted fate too much with his neglect of his health for all those years. Ironically, he decided to quit smoking to keep up with the increased oxygen demands of his new life with his new wife. At the time, he was already up to a pack a day even with his heart condition. When you quit after many years of smoking and your heart is so severely damaged, your body may no longer be able to deal with the detoxing. He died shortly after quitting smoking, right in the doctor's office. I always felt there was so much he could have done to help his own health and it broke my heart to lose my brother in his prime. Don't be like Bob. Don't wait until it is too late to help yourself. Don't tempt fate because you never know what the future may hold for you. You have so many resources to help restore, renew and regenerate your health. All you need is the knowledge and wisdom to get there.

I have been a Certified Ayurvedic Consultant since 2017 and have been involved with yogic sciences for over 20 years as of the writing of this book. In this time, I have seen how this knowledge transforms people's lives and helps them to be at their healthy best. I founded Susan Coach in 2015 as an educational company to help people achieve balanced health through exercises designed to boost the energy systems in their body and through nutritional knowledge that supports their growth at a cellular level.

I have seen incredible results for clients with this knowledge. My client Marietta had been suffering from inflammation in her body that showed up in her blood test results. It was creating neurological problems for her and was interfering with her quality of life. Her blood results had revealed that she had high liver enzymes, and her cardiac markers were also askew, including her C-reactive protein. She was nervous about her health and after working with her in tandem with an Ayurvedic physician she was able to change her blood results in two months with Ayurvedic remedies. We recommended immune-boosting herbal formulas and other remedies that were tailored for her dosha. Changing your health can be much simpler when you have the right tools. Ayurvedic tools focus a lot on cellular regeneration and nourishing the various systems of the body.

Cellular nutrition and detoxing are often overlooked in modern medicine, and the word "detox" has been misused so much that many nutritional consultants are choosing not to use the word at all. But here is the thing: gentle detoxing at the cellular level by Ayurvedic remedies and recipes can heal you at levels deeper than you can imagine. They are also easy to implement when you have the right teacher. The cells need oxygen and nutrients that will enhance cellular growth and not hinder it. Additives, sugars, unnecessary fats and GMOs are hidden in so many of our foods that it is hard to shop intelligently, even in natural health food stores. Taking too many supplements is never a good thing either. We will look at the hidden ingredients to avoid when shopping "natural" and how to create a lifestyle that supports natural health and beauty care. We will also learn the right rhythm and times of day to eat, exercises that boost instead of block your energies, and how to support the people you care about who may be experiencing health issues.

I first discovered Ayurveda when I was at a famous yoga center in the southern United States about 12 years ago. There was an Ayurvedic physician visiting from New York who was giving daily lectures on his book and the lectures were amazing. He talked about the toxins that naturopathic doctors were finding in the foods we eat. He talked about the dangers of plastics in our oceans which end up in our food and our bodies. This was throwing off our hormonal balance. He also talked about the recycling of prescription drugs that end up in our water supply that are wreaking havoc with our immune systems and hormonal levels. Wow, so much to digest here, no pun intended!

I went on to get trained as a Certified Ayurvedic Practitioner at a well-established institute in Manhattan, and this became an adjunct to my years of practice and study in the yogic sciences. This allowed me to speak firsthand to actual local physicians who were attending the class and having great results with their patients and their own health. As I learned about the doshas (the constitutions) of the body types and all the energy systems of the body (including *marma* points) and other more intricate subtle energy systems, I became intrigued. All my previous knowledge in the yogic sciences of health had just been verified. There was a clinical aromatherapist at the training who was taking an incredibly deep dive into the healing applications of essential oils. She was healing herself and her clients. I learned about the engagement of the *five senses* in the Ayurvedic healing process (sight, touch, sound, smell and taste) that all seemed to make such good sense. In Ayurveda there are *5 elements:* (earth, fire, air, water and ether) and each dosha is made up of two of them. During my Ayurvedic training, physicians and practitioners were achieving outstanding results with their clients and their own health. Many questions came up as I went through the process. For example, you may learn you have a fatty liver, but how do you heal it? Can you take a deeper dive to heal it with the proper nutrients and detoxing without overloading the system? Gooseberry, for example, a gentle supplement called *amalaki* and *shilajit* worked very well for a client I consulted with a fatty liver.

As you find out all the hidden gems of Ayurveda you will be able to enjoy the following benefits:

- feel more energy from the foods you eat
- feel rejuvenated as more oxygen nourishes your cells and your mind
- discover physical exercises that are creative and restore your health and energy
- easily incorporate essential oils and natural beauty care into your daily life
- learn how to add healing herbs and tonics to your daily routine
- naturally detox your cells and create a more alkaline body

One of the basic premises of health that Ayurvedic healing focuses on is the concept of the 7 Dhatus. Dhatu in Sanskrit means "element" or "constituent principle" and literally refers to the "stuff" of which our bodies are made. The 7 Dhatus in Ayurvedic medicine are:

1. Rasa Dhatu: Plasma tissue

2. Rakta Dhatu: Blood tissue
3. Mamsa Dhatu: Muscle tissue
4. Meda Dhatu: Fat Tissue
5. Asthi Dhatu: Bone Tissue
6. Majja Dhatu: Nerve and Bone Marrow Tissue
7. Shura Dhatu: Reproductive Tissue

Here is a picture of the 7 Dhatus:

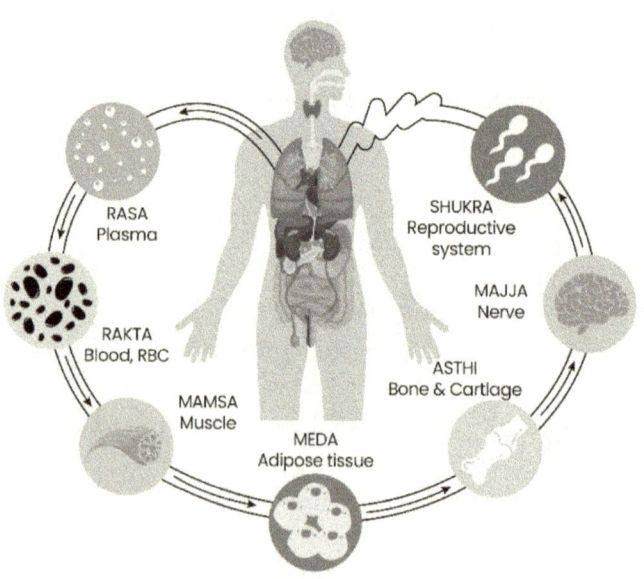

Ayurveda treats the whole person, and the support of the relationship between these 7 systems is the chief goal. A part cannot be separated from the whole, or you may miss the root cause. Rebalancing the 7 Dhatus is an integral part of Ayurvedic medicine.

When you open your mind to the benefits of Ayurveda, I hope you will want to share this information with the people that you care about. That is my big wish here. When you see people suffering or giving up, refer them to a trusted Ayurvedic professional and share the knowledge that you have learned with them too. Learning effective ways to share with people you care about is part of the magic of Ayurveda.

Once you start implementing the new knowledge that you are acquiring from Ayurveda you will be feeling more energized and balanced. You will find that it is the gift that keeps giving! You will always have a new herb, spice or essential oil to discover that will benefit your health and the health of the people you care about. As you continue to learn about all the exotic plants, oils and herbs in Ayurveda you will realize that you have at your fingertips (for a fraction of the cost of a hospital visit) all the necessary tools to survive and thrive in an ever-changing environment. You will then be able to help your kids and relatives to be guided to make changes that will impact their health and energy. You will truly be empowered with the wisdom of Ayurveda, and no one can take that away from you. You will be creating incredible health benefits that are measurable and will have your friends talking about the new you.

CHAPTER 2

Realize the Value of Your Health

When you realize the value of taking your health in your own hands, you empower yourself on so many levels. Don't be like Jessica, a dear family friend. She waited until it was too late and regretted not being able to watch her kids grow up and get married because of poor choices. Oh, it's easy to let the daily chore of caring for your health in a big way slip into the wrong hands. It happens from the moment you wake up in the morning until you go to bed in the evening every day. There are missed opportunities to feel better during every waking moment. Once you start making conscious choices for everything you do that align perfectly with the core principles of Ayurvedic wisdom, you will start feeling more energized and healthier. This is priceless.

The alcoholic drink you could have avoided, the checkup you never got, the things you could have done to prepare yourself mentally for the day's challenges never happened. Why? There will always be daily challenges. You may wake up feeling tired but don't know that with a few simple breathing exercises and a few essential oils you can change your state and feel energized. Jessica woke up feeling tired most days and then felt overwhelmed by the tasks at hand. This created a nervous dependency on a reckless routine and her mind was never at peace. She was smoking two packs of cigarettes a day. She knew she needed to quit smoking, but she had come to rely on the habit as a crutch. As she approached her early 50s, which we call *vata* age in Ayurveda, her health issues started to present as high blood pressure and eventually the big "C," cancer. She developed lung cancer and was starting to lose her voice. She finally knew she needed to quit, so she cut down instead of quitting entirely. She had let her health go so far, she truly believed she was past the point of no return.

The sad part is doctors had been telling her all along that it wasn't too late to take charge of her health, but she would have to admit that she had a problem. Then she would need to commit to a healthy solution that would make her feel better after she sufficiently detoxed her system from the smoking. All these years she was handing over her health to a cigarette company that cared nothing about her and that lured her into believing a cigarette would help her. Eventually it was too late, and she had to have a tracheotomy and she lost her voice permanently. Jessica was a dear family friend and is still struggling with the choices she made. She spends more time treating her condition than enjoying the years she has left. Just know that now is the best time to implement changes that will help you to restore, rejuvenate and regenerate your health with Ayurveda. This knowledge will support you during every step of your health journey.

I know you think you already know the right things to do to lead a healthy life, but there may be something stopping you from taking deliberate action on this. Health needs to be a priority, or it will start to retaliate against the neglect. Most people know they need to work out and to do both strength and cardiovascular training to be in top shape for their age and wellness category. They also know they need to avoid unhealthy additives in the foods they see on the grocery shelves and to be mindful of their digestion and absorption of nutrients. But for some reason they feel it becomes "too hard" or simply too much effort to keep up with. When you can calm the nervous energy of the mind (through mood-enhancing and meditative Ayurvedic techniques), you will start to see more clearly and wish you had known about this when you were a little kid.

Don't get stuck in the routine of being lazy in order to escape from your job, your responsibilities and/or life itself. It's your life and in the game of life, don't let the game win. Don't give away your confidence in your ability to empower your health to companies outside of yourself. From prescription meds to overloading on supplements, pick your poison. We are on information overload when it comes to the proper nutrition, exercise and lifestyle choices for our individual dosha. We are being hypnotized by packaged processed foods, "do it for you" ideas of fitness, and prescription pills to take away the problem. This is the easy way out and only focuses on the symptoms and not the root cause, as any natural healthcare provider will tell you. It's time to get your power back before it's too late.

Don't let your A-G-E-N-D-A get in the way. This is my acronym for what stops you from being proactive with your health so that you can be at your best. Don't let your A-G-E-N-D-A control you. It stands for:

A is *Acceptance*. You accept average health and don't care if your daily habits are taking away from your health. This is the reason that juvenile and adult obesity rates are off the charts in the U.S. We are not paying attention to what is important to our inner wellbeing. We are being taught that rich, fatty foods will make us happy. Supersize me! Or that you are one pill away from the promised land for your depression. Your depression is happening in your mind because you are not at peace with who you are and why you are here.

G is *Genetics*. You say it's in your genes. Your health woes are just your genes expressing themselves and even though this is at play, you can still improve your health in many, many ways. Don't give in to empowering the fact that a father, mother or some other blood relative had high cholesterol so therefore you are destined to deal with it. It's your vital organs and your diet; it's time to do something "restorative" instead of "reactive" to heal this condition.

E is for *Ego*. Your ego stops you from wanting to learn things that will enhance and optimize your health; drop it! It is never too late to learn something new that has been passed down for centuries, a system designed to support optimum health and performance. There is so much research out there to back this up, that now you do not have an excuse not to learn about it. You won't see this on TV or social media unless Ayurvedic consultants and physicians are talking about it there.

N is for *No time*. You believe you have no time to add Ayurvedic health tips into your day when just the opposite is true. It's easy to add to your daily routine and you will have more energy as you do it, so you will feel like there is more time in the day. Let that one go! You can just effortlessly add Ayurvedic health tips to your existing routine and have them become normal. You will start to notice a rhythm of how this all flows together naturally.

D is thinking that *detoxing is difficult*, and you think you don't even know where to begin. It's much easier than you think, and the detoxing happens gently in Ayurveda with guidance. Here we are talking about detoxing at the cellular level and, when done properly, is always achieved with gentle effective remedies. The remedies will restore balance to your cellular energy and metabolism and enhance your total health.

A is for *Avoiding* change. Here you may be avoiding changing your health habits as you go through life, until eventually it catches up to you. Don't be like Jessica and don't you dare be like Bob! Be flexible and embrace positive change! We are all changing right now, transforming, and now is the time to create incredible health and wellness.

When you avoid change and accept mediocrity in your health, you have cheated your own natural health birthright, and your body will start fighting back against you. Any successful system of health and wellness should be adaptable for a modern lifestyle. In Ayurveda you won't need to become vegetarian or vegan unless you want to, but you will be able to nourish, balance and cleanse your health on a very deeply energizing level. You will sleep better and be able to concentrate more. You will choose exercise routines that work for your dosha and the best times of day to eat so that you can properly absorb your food. This will empower you to create a healthy routine that is harmonious for your digestion and absorption of nutrients. You will discover the best types of foods, herbs, spices and natural care products that will support your own unique dosha.

Don't wait until your health starts acting up and miss out on a golden opportunity. It will still be there when you fall into despair, but why wait until then? When you avoid being proactive about your health you give in to the negative health programming that is all around us. This negative programming is in the media that you are constantly being exposed to! It's in the status reports of air and water quality in your environment. It's in the mortality stats from people who could have helped their health, had they acted sooner. It's in a belief system that you have that you don't have control over your health and wellness. That *you* don't matter, that *you* are not important enough. Remember health is true wealth. You can't take money and possessions with you when you go, and if you want to live a longer, healthier life, then you can't afford to sit back and do nothing! At the rate toxins are going into food, air and water supplies, we need all the natural ammunition we can get. Health is truly wealth and Ayurveda shows the way to lasting health. Ayurveda includes exercise, nutrition, herbs, spices, essential oils and breathing exercises that will support you through life's seasons.

Take, for example, my client David. He took action on his health during the direst of times. He was 52 years old at the time and new to Ayurveda. He had been starting to enjoy the food and the routine when Covid hit him hard. Here he did have genetic markers that did not favor a successful recovery as he was very sick with pneumonia. But he avoided being intubated and put on a ventilator and was catheterized instead. As he started to recover from the Covid, his body went into diabetes. There were genetic markers in his family history for diabetes and high cholesterol. He fought through a tough mindset and pulled through the Covid only to deal with the diabetes. It was tough for him to experience the onset of what was termed full-blown diabetes by his doctor. Rather than freaking out, he looked at his A1C and thought: "What can I do to get out of this mess? If I keep going on like this, I won't be here for my kids' milestones." He was 5'10" and 250 pounds at the time and managed to lose 80 pounds with his own belief in being in charge of his health. He knew that weight loss would help and it only took him 8-12 weeks to achieve, which is stunning. Sadly, being sick helped him drop weight too.

He applied what he had learned in Ayurveda to ingest the right herbs, spices and nutrients that he knew would support a healthy blood sugar level as he dropped the extra pounds. Human physiology is complex, and we need to rely on our allopathic physicians for the statistics and blood results, and, from there we can take constructive action. This is exactly what David did in an incredible way. I can't take credit for his transformation as he did this mostly on his own, but I can humbly say the empowerment he received from learning Ayurveda enhanced his own rock-steady dosha, which for David was *Pitta* or fire. Pitta is one of the three constitutions in Ayurveda and it is a fiery one.

The first stage in learning about Ayurveda is understanding the three doshas and the context in which the word dosha is being used. For basic knowledge of Ayurveda, it's good to know that these words come from Sanskrit. A good working knowledge of the Sanskrit terms will be enlightening. Please see the glossary at the end of this book. It will help you as you read it. For understanding the doshas it is helpful to know that here the term is being used to describe your body and personality type. The three dosha types in this context are *pitta* (fire), *kapha* (earth) and *vata* (air). There are seven possible doshas because there are combinations of the three, which will be described in the next chapter.

The next stage in Ayurveda is learning about the five elements that are used to describe the doshas, and they are air, ether, water, fire and earth. Each of the dosha types are made up of two elements, and that describes their general nature. So just remember pitta, kapha and vata and the five elements according to Ayurveda and you will be on your way to understanding body types and personalities. Here dosha means your bioenergetics and general personality. These terms will also be used to describe health problems in certain areas of the body too. You will discover the nature of human health and cellular activity from an Ayurvedic perspective and it is fascinating stuff!

The reason I feel that now is the best time to start learning about Ayurveda is that I have seen too many people (mostly family members) who have given in to poor health. Some developed adult-onset diabetes, others needed triple bypass surgery, and many unfortunately passed away too soon. Their own poor health could have been corrected by applying these principles and taking charge of their health. They didn't have to give their health power away. Don't be like the ones we have lost along the way, who have allowed co-morbidities to develop in their bodies by neglecting their weight, eating habits, exercise habits and mental outlook. Don't fall into the "Someday I'll" Club where you fill in the blanks. Someday I'll make time for self-care when I am not working so much; someday I'll take better care of my health when I change my job, etc. It's like saving for your health future the way you would save for your financial future. You don't want to go into your future broke from a health standpoint, do you? Then what will you do? Choose the "health is wealth" way that Ayurveda provides and you will have peace of mind.

The good news is that the population at large is starting to wake up to natural health benefits and the sense of well-being that Ayurveda can bestow upon a person if they take the time to understand its concepts. It's important that Ayurveda is explained in a way that is not so lofty and exclusive. The joys and wonders of Ayurvedic wisdom need to be made inclusive and accessible for everyday understanding and application. Then incredible transformation can happen because it will be more accessible for the masses.

✦ *Think you are too old or green to benefit from the incredible health perks of Ayurveda?*

People of all ages can start reaping the benefits right away. Kids can start eating healthy snacks at school and applying some of the concepts around sleep time and melatonin production that will enhance their wellbeing. Adults at any age can start feeling relief from inflammatory conditions, digestive issues and general adrenal fatigue.

✦ *Worried you don't have enough time in the day to make these changes?*

Ayurveda health tips can slide easily into your day and will only enhance it. You will become more aware of your eating, sleeping and exercise habits than ever before so you will start to make those areas perform more efficiently for you. For example, scheduling exercises into an existing routine that is tailored to your nervous system will give you more energy and clarity throughout the day. When it comes to sleep routine, less is more so you can start subtracting distractions like electronics and mind chatter after a certain hour of the night to allow your nervous system to sync with your brain for deeper, more regenerative sleep.

✦ *Are you thinking it's too hard to learn or to create healthy changes?*

Remember that any successful health system (especially one that has been on the planet for centuries and most likely thousands of years) should have an implementation plan that is simple and adaptable to a modern lifestyle. The true beauty in Ayurveda is in the simplicity of applying it to what you are already doing. So, you add a new tea to your routine, and you see how it's helping you, you add a few spices and a few grains to your foods, and you start to notice your digestion has improved. You can easily move away from eating on the run and recognize the smartest times of day to eat for better digestion and stoking of your digestive fire (or *agni* in Sanskrit).

◆ *Think it's difficult to find the ingredients and the spices and all the other Ayurvedic goodies?*

Fear not, because you can find them in most cities, or they can be easily ordered, and you will see that they are affordable too. Many Indian food stores and some grocery and specialty stores carry Ayurvedic products that are easy to find. Create your own Golden Milk as a delicious night drink with easy to find spices and ingredients like turmeric and coconut milk. Looking for natural hygiene products? These days you can find Vicodent, a natural Ayurvedic toothpaste that strengthens your gums and Neem, a refreshing natural facial cleanser that feels great on the skin. Neem is in most Indian stores and some natural health food stores. There are a number of stores that sell online and when you are buying herbs, grains, spices or essential oils, you will see that they are very affordable too! Saffron is a little expensive but totally worth it, and remember health is true wealth.

◆ *Concerned you won't be able to stick to it?*

You will find it enjoyable and easy to apply to what you are already currently doing; that is the point of making Ayurveda accessible. When you enjoy what you are doing and it is being taught to you in an easy to access way, you can enjoy the health benefits and that will motivate you. You will find you can naturally stay away from chemicals and additives in your foods and hygiene products. Your senses will be heightened, and this will motivate you to keep going because you will be enjoying the process.

When I had my first consultation with an Ayurvedic expert a number of years ago, she discovered that I had an underactive thyroid. I felt fine and had no health concerns, although I did have trouble losing weight. The Ayurvedic physician had taken my pulse, looked at the whites of my eyes and had asked detailed questions about my digestion and absorption of nutrients, my sleep and exercise habits, and overall wellness. She was able to detect those subtle yet accurate imbalances in my life and this allowed me to enhance my own health. My underactive thyroid did not warrant traditional medicine as it appeared to be a correctable metabolic issue. This is a common diagnosis for many people. Since Ayurvedic remedies are individualized, it will be custom tailored to your own unique body and dosha. The supplements recommended to me were easy on my system and were made from pure ingredients that were designed to support and restore my thyroid. They were immune system boosting and many of them were simple foods that I added to my diet. Within a few weeks of taking these gentle remedies and adding the foods, I started to feel lighter and healthier. I could sense a change was happening.

Over time, this made it easier for me to lose weight and I discovered I had more energy. These were all indicators that my health was moving in the right direction. And when I spoke to an NYC physician who was in my NYC Ayurvedic graduate training class, she reported that she had a similar condition to mine (thyroid and metabolic in nature) and had achieved incredible results with following an Ayurvedic protocol that was tailored for her unique health. The results that I have received from clients and colleagues have been no less than outstanding, and I know that you can have the same results when you embrace it.

When you tap into the knowledge of Ayurveda and use the principles to take charge of your health you will notice feelings of wellbeing and glowing health. You will want to share with your friends, family, colleagues, and students. The more we can spread the word about the incredible health benefits in a way that is accessible to everyone, the more it will be in vogue. Imagine being able to create an organic face wash and toner from items you have in your own fridge. Or to boost your immune system with a simple three-ingredient tea that is easy to make with things you can buy from your local grocery store. Or a two-ingredient essential oil facial sauna that you can put together in minutes with a saucepan and a towel that will open up your airways and sinuses! The list goes on and on. When you realize that the love and joy of healthy natural living with Ayurveda is at your fingertips, you can truly smile as you embrace this for many years to come. It's incredible to think of how vast a field of study it is and that there will always be things to learn. We are using this knowledge as a complementary natural approach to boost your health and wellness in a meaningful way for many years to come. It is truly the gift that keeps giving.

CHAPTER 3

Get to Know Ayurveda

These days, amidst all the noise and haste and conflicting opinions, there is hope for you to take exquisite command of your health. Ayurveda gives you simple yet sophisticated tools to make your modern lifestyle simply healthier. The cool thing is that you can grow healthier year after year as you integrate the fun, easy-to-do methods here that make it accessible for you. One of my clients was so impressed with the natural skincare methods of Ayurveda that she eventually became an aesthetician and started teaching others how to naturally take care of their skin. While she was treating clients to her facials, she would pamper them with beautiful rose hips, chamomile and lavender. When she started learning about the simple ingredients she could find around the house for natural skincare, she became unstoppable.

Another client started experimenting with different recipes in order to integrate Ayurvedic herbs, foods and spices into her kids' meals. She found they enjoyed the meals more and she never mentioned a word about what she was doing. She noticed her kids were healthier and less hyper and she attributed this to the good nutritional value her kids were getting from the meals. She even noticed that the reduction in sugar and additive intake made them feel calmer and happier. Let's face it, you are what you eat, and Ayurveda gives a great roadmap for success.

Here are seven things to know about Ayurveda, and they are all easy to start integrating into your lifestyle. When you use them, you will notice that they will enhance your natural vitality and give you incredible hope. You can start relieving your body from inflammation and subtle destructive forces that are present in the foods and products you use. This includes mental inflammation, which is present in the types of things we read, hear and see every day. You will learn tools that improve the quality of your life on so many levels; from your sleep patterns and home environment to the times of day and quality of foods that you eat. You can also create a community of likeminded people around this idea if you want to. In Ayurveda we engage all the senses (sight, sound, taste, touch and smell) through the remedies. You will find yourself engaged in this new lifestyle that you are creating. Let the fun begin!

7 Things to Know About Ayurveda:

1. Know Your Dosha and Make It Work for You

One of your many health assets from Ayurveda will be knowing your dosha. Remember, we are using dosha to describe your general personality and bioenergy as opposed to using dosha (pitta, kapha, vata) to describe a health problem in the body. Your dosha is based upon the three types: fire (pitta), earth (kapha) and air (vata) and there are seven possible dosha types since you can be a combination of two doshas or three doshas (tridoshic). When you know your dosha type, you will have insights into the types of exercise, foods, daily routines and skin care that will work best for you. You will have insights into your unique, natural tendencies and energies, and this will help guide you into making more creative choices when it comes to enhancing your health. We will go over how to test for your dosha and will explore what works best for you. Most people are a combination of two doshas and some can be a combo of all three (tridoshic), so in total there are seven combinations. Which one are you?

The seven dosha types and their combinations are:

- Vata
- Pitta
- Kapha
- Vata Pitta
- Pitta Kapha
- Vata Kapha
- Vata Kapha Pitta

The proportions of the doshas will also vary from one individual to the next, and this will allow you to get very specific about your health if that is your goal. At that level, your Ayurvedic knowledge will become a superpower.

2. Exercise for Your Dosha

Modern-day exercise classes are more of a one size fits all and they may not always benefit your spinal health and the energy systems in your body. You will learn which ones benefit your dosha and this will help to balance your energy. Since Ayurveda is a complete system of health that looks at the whole person, you may find that certain types of calisthenics and even yoga classes may be aggravating instead of enhancing your health. You will discover how to differentiate between the ones that are helping and those that are not helping at all. Yoga exercises and stretches can easily be incorporated into your daily routine. This will help you to know the best types of exercises that you should be doing. You can even start to integrate a few exercises at home that can strengthen your spine and balance your neurology.

This type of knowledge can be a blessing during times of stress and fatigue while traveling around and around on the wheel of life. Life can bring so many responsibilities and modern-day burdens. You can tap into these simple stretches that activate your spine and regenerate your health. These exercise tips, tricks and hacks can be a godsend when you crave a much-needed pick-me-up. Learn to use them and appreciate their simplicity and you will be well on your way to empowering your body and your mind (your body/mind) for healthy success.

3. Breathing Exercises / Pranayama for Your Dosha

Pranayama, or breathing exercises that derive from yoga tradition, are hidden gems that most people do not even know how to use for practical everyday living. There are many types of breathing exercises that can be broken down into simple elements: breath retention (gently holding your breath for a certain length of time), breath exhalation (one main goal is to develop a long exhalation) and breath bellows (a panting-like gesture) designed to expel stale air and to rejuvenate the belly or throat area depending on how it is done. Just know that these exercises can be very easy to add to your day and they can be huge stress relievers. They can certainly change your state of mind at any given moment, if used properly.

In modern-day coaching, therapy and the arts, everyone is reminded to breathe. How did we forget such a basic function and why are we having trouble adding breathing to our day? This may be because we live in the western world and tend to be in our heads most of the time. We seem to be spending less time in our bodies. When you get out of your head and into your body, you will find it is so simple that you may think it's too easy. Then you can allow your own breath to be there for you like a lifelong friend. After all, your breath is with you for life. It needs acknowledgment and you can harness it to serve you.

4. Transform Your Kitchen / Know Your Herb, Spice and Plant Friends

They say home is where the heart is, and Ayurveda agrees. How does your kitchen look now? Is it warm and inviting and is there space to cook and organize? Don't be worried if it is not, as modern living has sometimes made the kitchen less of a thing. However, post-pandemic, people started to tune into the joys of cooking and gathering around the kitchen. Let's go that route and start to learn about the most commonly used spices in Ayurveda. You can also learn about some herbs, spices and plants you may never have heard of that are excellent for your health. Health begins with getting to know these herbs, spices and plants and organizing them properly in your home. They will be your best friends and will help you digest and absorb your food. Many of the common ones you know, like garlic, ginger and turmeric, have anti-microbial and anti-fungal properties that are stellar for your health.

Ayurveda teaches us that we are being bombarded daily by allergens, viruses and bacteria, and that we need the proper tools in the form of nutrition, remedies and lifestyle changes to combat these daily stressors. These days we are becoming more aware of this as the microbiome or gut health is finally being taught a little by modern medicine. In that way, allopathic medicine is just starting to catch up to what Ayurveda has been teaching for thousands of years.

5. Know Your Foods that Aid Digestion / Best Times of Day for Digesting

One coping mechanism that people have caught onto in modern living is the concept of comfort eating and rewarding themselves with food. This contributes to obesity and can easily set someone up for pre-diabetes/diabetes. The comfort food may be tasty but does little to strengthen your health. When you start to tune into your body's digestion and absorption patterns you will start to look at food and eating differently. You will start to crave healthy foods more and see the comfort foods for what they truly are: dead foods that are stripping your health away, slowly but surely. As Ayurvedic practitioners we ask you detailed questions about your digestion and absorption of nutrients so that we can help you choose more wisely the times of day that you eat and the types of foods you should be preferring. You will become more aware of your eating routine and how you feel afterward. When you start to add Ayurvedic tips to your everyday routine, you will be rewarded by having more energy to carry out your daily life in style. We do live in a stressful world, and we tend to worry about the future. We should claim our birthright to be living, eating, and breathing at our best every day. Why settle for anything less? Since when did disease become a focal point of health in our society? Why not focus on what to do to create optimum health? It's time to take back the reins of health instead of living in fear about what can happen. Ayurveda shows the way.

6. Yoga Nidra / Sleep Patterns / Decompress from the Day

Ever notice that your cell phone light seems glaring when you are looking at it in bed? Or that your mind can't seem to turn off at night? Some people leave lights on and a movie playing in the background in order to fall asleep. No, no, no! This does nothing to regenerate the body and the mind. You need to experience the natural rejuvenation that a good night's sleep can afford. A good night's sleep can be your greatest ally and will restore your health and repair your body if you let it. You will need all the help that you can get, and Ayurveda has some ideas that will help you so much. Guided meditation as you drift off in the form of yoga nidra will enhance your night's sleep and will transfer your thinking from mind chatter into mind calm.

Natural melatonin forms in the presence of darkness, which is why it is important for it to be dark (with all electronics off) when dozing off at night. If you have trouble sleeping, you will find that some of the breathing and physical exercises can help your body feel naturally tired at night. The atmosphere of your room, the sounds in the background and the position you sleep in are all at play. Add some soothing essential oils, practice some *marma* (Ayurvedic pressure points) release and practice sleeping in the dark. This will enhance your overall wellbeing. You will awaken feeling refreshed and regenerated. More on this later.

7. Know Marma Energy Points / Receive Ayurvedic Massage with Marma Points

The energy points in the body in Ayurveda are both internal and external. They operate on some very subtle channels that can be used to strengthen the immune system and to energize the body/mind. *Marma points* are key energy points on your body that can help you do self-massage and can also be applied during a regular massage. Knowledge and stimulation of these energy points can restore balance to the body. You can think of them as energy channels or *nadis* that are connected to all your organs, your nervous system and your vital energy or *prana*. The study of marma points may predate that of acupuncture as it goes back literally thousands of years.

For our intention of keeping this simple and accessible, these energy points tend to move in an upward location and are more circular than linear in nature. As you discover their connecting points on the body, you will be able to give self-massage when areas of your body seem a little tired. You can also treat yourself to an Ayurvedic massage where essential oils and herbs can be used to heal your body to an exquisite level. Ayurvedic massage can energize your body on a deep level, while nourishing your cells and enhancing your dosha. There are a number of different types of massage that you can order when you go to an Ayurvedic center. My personal favorite is *abyanga*, a full-body massage, although *Shirodhara* (head massage) can be highly beneficial for other things a person may have going on. In Ayurveda, there is always something going on with your health and it's good to catch it before it has a chance to develop into anything serious. Here is the fundamental difference between treating disease (the basic premise of western medicine) and enhancing health.

The beauty of putting all these healthy aspects of an Ayurvedic lifestyle together is that we can create our health as we like it. We don't have to be subject to someone else's idea of how our health is to be. Let's face it, we can be so much more than simply in a state of "preventing or managing a disease." We can move into a gracious state of truly restoring our health on a joyous level. Why not enjoy our health while we have it and embrace more fully the life we have been given? If we can share this knowledge with the people we care about, we can create a community that has a healthy outlook on life.

When you think of what this can do for the youth or seniors of tomorrow, there can be the promise of a brighter, much healthier future than we have ever imagined. We can help those we care about who have an over reliance on prescription pills. Or those people who hand over their health to someone outside of themselves. In America, we have had it wrong for too long with fast foods and fast health fixes. This has been a contributing factor to the rising levels of heart disease and diabetes in this country. It's time to start fighting back in a smart way that will boost a healthy lifestyle.

CHAPTER 4

Know Thy Constitution or Dosha

> *"A person's cells will start to take on unique characteristics from the time of conception, according to Ayurveda. This will develop into your dosha where dosha refers to your bioenergy and general personality traits."*
>
> – Susan Holman

According to Ayurvedic texts, the moment you were conceived, your cells started to differentiate and create the unique configuration that is you! You can thank the ovum and the sperm of your biological parents for how you became you. It runs deep as any ancient wisdom philosophy that was handed down by the sages of old. But basically, the moment you were conceived, your cells started differentiating to form your internal organs, your brain, your blood and bones and the energy running through them. So, the "deep" idea is that cellular nutrition and cleansing can create incredible results in healing your body/mind from within.

This chapter will give you insights into the three basic constitutional components in Ayurveda:

pitta (fire), *kapha* (earth) and *vata* (air) and the five elements (air, space, fire, water and earth). Each dosha is made up of two elements. You will see how they describe your unique characteristics in terms of energy, personality and health. There are a total of seven dosha types because a person is usually a combination of 1-2 doshas. When we as Ayurvedic experts check your health by asking questions, taking your pulse and understanding how you digest and absorb your food, a pattern will be revealed and your dosha will be described in one of the following seven constitutional types:

- *Pitta*
- *Kapha*
- *Vata*
- *Vata-Pitta*
- *Pitta -Kapha*
- *Vata-Kapha*
- *Vata-Kapha-Pitta. Or Tri-Dosha*

You can see them below in a chart.

As mentioned before, in Ayurveda the constitutions are made up of five elements, space, air, water, fire, and earth. (This is different from the five elements in Chinese medicine. In Chinese medicine they swap out air and space for metal and wood. It appears that Ayurveda predates Chinese medicine.) Knowing the five elements in Ayurveda will help you know how to understand your dosha more fully. A pattern will emerge, and it will help you plan your health strategy in a way that boosts your immune system and regenerates your internal health. Let's explore which of the five elements are in each dosha. Knowing your dosha type and the elements that are present in each one will help you to understand your health's characteristics.

The two elements that make up each dosha:

- *Vata is composed of air and space.*
- *Kapha is composed of water and earth.*
- *Pitta is composed of water and fire.*

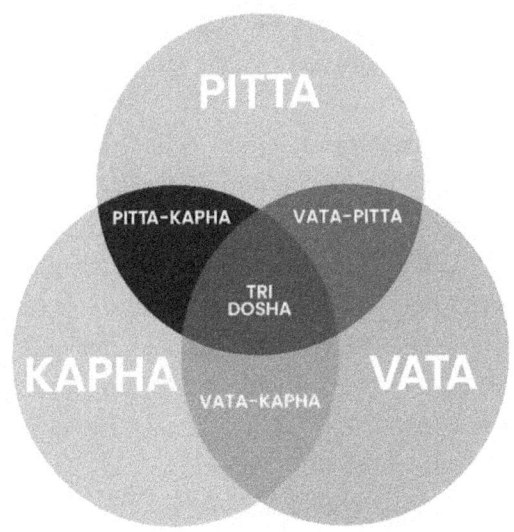

When treating your dosha, foods and exercise can be prescribed to enhance your energy body and boost your health. Let's look at the characteristics of the doshas and then you can start to see what traits you share with them.

This chart shows the basic types:

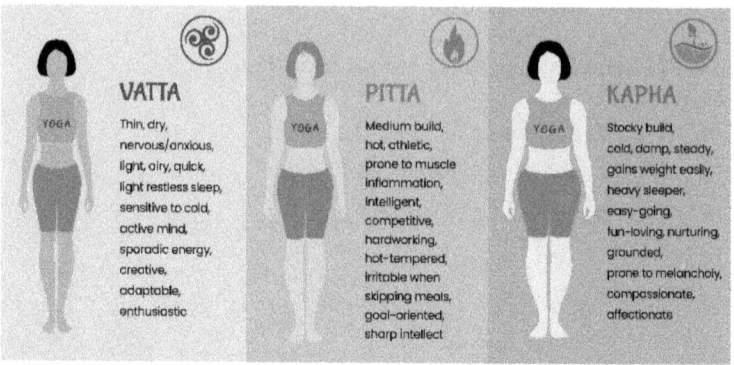

Here you can see how your body type and tendencies will describe other areas of your health. These are similar on the surface to Sheldon's system of endomorph (round fat type), mesomorph (muscular type) and ectomorph (skinny, slim type). You have to ask where Sheldon may have gotten his body type information from. The difference between a basic body type classification and Ayurveda is that Ayurveda will take these many levels deep in the body into tissue, digestion, blood, bone and organ health. In Ayurvedic medicine, the "stuff" of which bodies are made is very important and will be governed by the basic dosha for the individual.

Let's look at the five elements of Ayurveda and how they relate to each basic dosha:

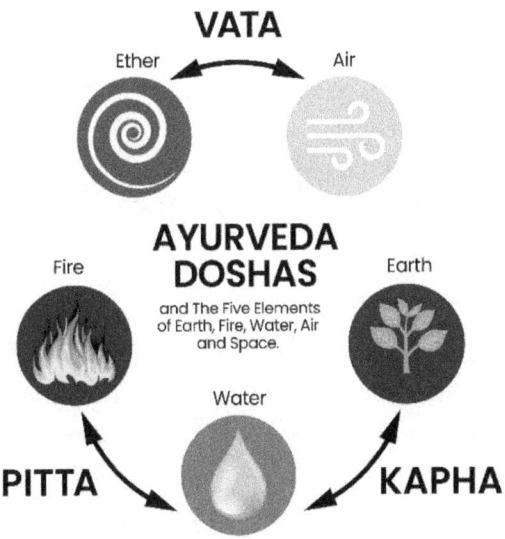

I know I am throwing a lot of beautiful Sanskrit terminology at you, but let's face it, it is so worth it when you start to understand this amazing system of health. How many health systems can you think of that teach you how to eat, exercise, sleep and do proper self-care to nourish your body, mind and soul from the inside out? How did this knowledge come into existence? Let me give you the short version and you can research the rest on your own. It is now time that the lofty ideals and health benefits of Ayurvedic wisdom become accessible for the everyday person and not just for people exposed to natural health alternatives and yogic science. Although this book is also for those people too!

Ayurvedic medicine has a rich history and was originally shared as an oral tradition. It was recorded more than 5,000 years ago in Sanskrit in the four sacred texts of the Vedas: the Rig Veda (3000-

2500 BCE), the Yajur Veda and Altharva Veda (1200-1000 BCE) and the Sam Veda. The initial offering of the knowledge was shared orally from the ancient seers or *rishis* of India. Ayurveda has been used extensively in clinical and natural health settings throughout the world and is only recently becoming popular in the U.S. Current knowledge about Ayurveda is primarily based on texts called the *Brhattrayi,* which consist of the *Charak Samhita, Sushurta Samhita* and *Ashtanga Hridaya.* These are some of the earliest known texts on surgery and medicine in the world which are incredibly specific.

Let's look at the doshas and see where you are on the Ayurvedic spectrum. *Kapha* (earth) dosha consists of a broad, strong curvy body type and gains weight easily with difficulty losing weight. The eyes tend to be rounded with a softer gaze. The skin tends to be oily, thick and cool and the hair is wavy, oily and thick. The *kapha* constitution tends to have a steady appetite and a calm, steady and grounded personality. The *kapha* speech is slow, deep, low and melodious and they tend to enjoy routine and also leisurely activity. Their sweat is moderate, and their process of elimination is slow, moderate and usually regular. Keep in mind that these are general characteristics that will make sense in the big picture of Ayurveda as we go along.

You can probably think of people you know like this who speak slowly, tend to take life in its stride, and are probably carrying a few extra pounds. From a neurological standpoint they tend to be relaxed in nature and this contributes to their longevity and makes them fun to be around. A *kapha* tends to put your mind at ease. Take, for example, my client Lucy, who is a *kapha/pitta* so she has two constitutions within her that can balance each other or can fight each other depending on what she has going on internally. For her the *kapha* gives a lightheartedness but also makes it difficult to lose weight. There is an art to losing weight when one is a *kapha* type and I will share more on this later. Exercise needs to be more intense but targeting areas specific to *kapha* type (where fat might accumulate easily).

Pitta (fire) dosha body type tends to be medium build and muscular. Although they can gain weight easily, it is also easy for them to lose it, and this becomes a metabolic trait of the *pitta* dosha. Their skin tends to be warm, oily, sunburns easily and sometimes they have freckles. Their hair is straight and fine and sometimes becomes gray early. Their eyes tend to be brightly colored with an intensity of gaze. The pitta appetite is intense, and they tend to sweat a lot. Their general temperament is bright, ambitious, driven and sometimes arrogant. They tend to dislike heat and humidity and are competitive and intense by nature. They tend to learn quickly and forget slowly, and their process of elimination is regular, loose and a large quantity. How many *pitta* types can you think of off the bat? All the constitutions run deep in the body and into the organs as well so there will be a lot to discover, and it will become much more specific. We do have an overrun of *pitta* types on the planet and it can generally be used to describe overly ambitious intense types with a strong gaze. It is made of fire and water, and it is usually the fire aspect that causes the *pitta* to overheat and burn out if not careful.

Vata (air) dosha tends to have a thin frame and tends to be skinny. They find it easy to lose weight and hard to gain it. We see this type a lot in runners. Their skin is cold, dry and thin and their hair also is thin, dry and sometimes frizzy. Their eyes tend to be small, and their appetite is irregular. Keep in mind, the *vata* dosha is made of both air and space elements and it shows in their focus and other aspects of their type. They learn quickly but tend to forget quickly as well and their speech is high-pitched, talkative and fast. They scarcely sweat. They tend to be scattered and it is difficult for them to focus when they are talking to you. Their appetite is irregular, and their process of elimination is dry, constipated, irregular and usually in small quantity. They are creative, energetic, nervous and indecisive. They tend to dislike routine and crave variety. They are restless, social and active. The airiness of *vata* dosha will usually need some grounding techniques for them to get focused and to ground their energy. The *vata's* airy and dry nature will need to be tended to in prescribing remedies.

How will understanding your dosha empower your health? You can think of it as a roadmap to living a healthy, long life. This roadmap is set with hidden treasures and gems along the way, which can help you navigate the occasional roadblocks that will come up in any health journey. Knowledge is power because we look at signals in Ayurvedic consultations that indicate that there may be toxicity or sluggishness in the system. The basic theory acknowledges that bacteria, viruses and fungi exist in your internal terrain, so just about everyone will have something "going on" with their health that they might not be aware of. Since most modern medicine deals with disease, Ayurveda affords you a great opportunity to catch things building up in your system early on, so that you will be way ahead of the game.

The more chemicals and pollutants that are introduced into our food and environment, the higher the chances are that we are dealing with something in our systems that can be detected during an Ayurvedic consultation. For the purpose of this book, I will be focusing on preventive applications that can save you time and energy. I will share preventive Ayurvedic diagnoses and remedies and case studies here. There is plenty of research on the medical applications for helping patients with disease and some will be cited in this book.

What are some things that an Ayurvedic consultation can detect that will help you on the road to regenerating your health? Some of the most common things detected are fatty liver, sluggish thyroid, and cholesterol and triglyceride problems. When we take your pulse, we are looking to see initially how it is running: is it running fast *(pitta)*, jumpy *(vata)* or sluggish *(kapha)*? If you are a *pitta* person with a *kapha* dominant pulse, something is sluggish in the system. We look at your tongue for the presence of *ama*, or toxicity. Ama is a toxic substance formed in the body due to poor digestion and metabolism. When the body's metabolism is compromised it makes ama to cause toxins to stick to the intestinal tract, to penetrate the skin cells, to clog arteries, and to fog the mind's nerve channels. It usually appears as a whitish coat on the tongue.

I am sure that you have heard of tongue scraping, which is a cleansing technique used in yoga to sweep the *ama* off the tongue. But we have a bigger problem than that. The presence of *ama* indicates metabolic and digestive inefficiencies that are compromising one's health. The microbiome is an integral part of Ayurvedic health remedies and, since there is a lot of conflicting information on the microbiome, it is best to adhere to the simplest, most natural remedies. Ayurvedic remedies can restore proper digestion and absorption of nutrients in the gut and ideally help you develop your own beneficial bacteria in the gut so that you can rely on your body's ability to heal itself.

My client Kathy came to me a few years ago. An Ayurvedic consultation clearly revealed the presence of *ama* and indicators of a fatty liver. Fatty liver is so common these days that most medical facilities are aware of it. When asked how to treat it, some natural healing doctors and practitioners recommend milk thistle and dandelion and these are both very good, but the real question to ask is how can I repair and restore my liver in order to start healing it from within without relying on so many supplements? Enter the detoxing lifestyle recommendations of Ayurveda that are all a part of this beautiful healthcare system. Here you will understand and empower your health through detoxing and intermittent fasting techniques that again are based on dosha.

I worked closely with Kathy, and we started her out with *amalaki* (gooseberry) and *shilajit* (a mineral pitch) and started to make gradual, easy-to-follow modifications to her diet. She was constantly eating on the run and her digestion fire or *agni* was burning out. There were increased levels of cortisol in her system that were naturally interfering with her body's ability to lose weight. When we realized the times of day that would be most beneficial for her to digest her food, we integrated intermittent fasting (for her that meant not eating after 7 or 8 p.m.) and her health started to improve rapidly. Intermittent fasting has been used in Ayurveda for thousands of years, and it will give your body a much-needed break from the bombardment of food, especially food eaten at the worst time for your digestive fire to kick in. Other remedies used to help detox and restore her liver included detox ghee, fasting smoothies and castor oil packs.

Once Kathy started to experience the gentle benefits of the Ayurvedic remedies, she started to notice a general sense of wellbeing and a calm she had never experienced before. She felt like she had control over her own health. We integrated the seven concepts for great health in Ayurveda mentioned in Chapter 3. Here's how they worked for Kathy:

- *Dosha Knowledge:* Through taking her pulse and understanding her dosha, Kathy was able to cool some *pitta* imbalances she was experiencing.
- *Exercise for Your Dosha:* She needed slower, more sustained yoga postures to be added to her ambitious *pitta*-driven exercise routine; she started noticing results right away! Her energies were more balanced, and her muscles felt relief from stress.

- *Breathing Exercises or Pranayama:* These Sanskrit words will save your life. We kept the breathing exercises gentle yet powerful for Kathy. Oxygen was able to reach her cells and free radicals in her system started to be destroyed. This worked very well for Kathy because we kept the exercises so simple, she could even do them on the train or in her cubicle at work!
- *Transform Your Kitchen / Know Your Herb, Spice and Plant Friends:* Kathy started to learn how much fun it can be to add these herbs and spices to her meals. These herbs, spices and plants quickly became her kitchen (and on-the-go) friends. She was able to throw together easy to prepare meals and to play with different creations.
- *Know Foods that Aid Digestive Fire / Best Times of Day to Eat:* Kathy became motivated by the extra energy she felt when she ate the right foods for her digestion. By fine-tuning her digestive *agni* she was able to perform at her best. She curbed cravings by having easy to prepare healthy snacks on hand. Giving her digestive fire the right breaks through intermittent fasting and Ayurvedic boosts, she became unstoppable!
- *Yoga Nidra / Sleep Patterns / Decompress from the Day:* Before she came to me, Kathy was waking up in the middle of the night with anxiety. As she shifted her diet naturally, she tuned into restoring herself through proper sleep and "unplugging." We did guided sleep meditation (yoga nidra) and enforced the habit of unplugging nightly so that her anxiety was replaced gradually by serenity.
- *Know Your Marma Energy Points / Receive Ayurvedic Massage with Marma Points:* Kathy had fun with this and benefitted from head massages, or *Shirodhara*, for the particular health issues she had going on. Her transformation has been very rewarding to watch as she shares what she has learned with her family. The yogic science that is the cornerstone of Ayurvedic health involves knowledge of energy points in the body for both self-massage, couples massage and

regular Ayurvedic massage treatments. This can be so regenerating and fun that it can be habit-forming. This is a good addiction to have!

Just ask yourself : *"How good am I willing to allow myself to feel?"* This is an age-old question and the yogis through time are telling us the sky is the limit. Just don't get so attached to this body that you lose sight of how to help others and the world around you. Even though the body is a temporary house for you for now, it would be smart to keep the house happy and balanced and looking its best. There are so many mixed messages out there when it comes to health that the world needs more healthy, vibrant people running around to help fix some of the toxic ideas that surround health in our world today. The notion of supersizing or throwing sugar and chemicals at our foods has been going on for many decades now. The dependence on Adderall, opioids and other prescription drugs has gotten out of control.

You can enhance your own knowledge of health with Ayurvedic lifestyle changes by adding a simple yearly blood test to your natural healing toolkit. You do not need to be a medical doctor to understand what your cholesterol, HDLs, LDLs, liver enzymes and complete blood count are. Have your primary care doctor interpret it but learn what you need to pay attention to, to energize your health and restore it. Want to know what your hormone panel is? Get a gender-based panel and see for yourself and compare it to the median levels. These days everyone is monitoring their A1C but what about actively lowering the numbers?

We have been led to believe that these numbers define us, but this cannot even be logically correct because every day our body is changing. Modern medicine is making breakthrough advances in colon and pancreatic health, even though it may seem slow in coming. Always ask: *"What can I do to increase my level of health and live my best life?"* You will find that you have more resources than you ever thought possible. There are an infinite number of Ayurvedic herbs, spices and remedies that will keep you busy for many lifetimes. You only need to know a few to get rid of *ama* and to boost your digestive *agni*. It doesn't involve a million supplements or the next shiny object when you have an early detection system like an Ayurvedic consultation. Ayurvedic knowledge will help you see where your body is holding toxicity. On top of this you won't be overloading your system (your poor liver) with endless supplements or the new flavor of the month. You will learn how to get back to the basics of natural healing with the idea that *less is more*. The beauty of this is that most herbal remedies and tonics in Ayurveda are very inexpensive. They are gentle in their application and their power resides in their restorative capacity.

I have heard in my Ayurvedic travels many success stories that will inspire you. I remember when I came across a famous Ayurvedic physician who has a practice in California who was helping a lady who had leaky bowel syndrome. Her malady was brought on by radiation therapy to help cure her uterine cancer. She was in her early 60s and, although her cancer was gone, the leaky bowel was becoming a very noticeable aftereffect from the radiation therapy. She couldn't attend classes publicly and the leaky bowel was an embarrassment. She started adhering to an Ayurvedic diet and used Ayurvedic herbal remedies that totally cured her when nothing else worked. Her routine and diet would have to be stricter than anything you would need to do in order to enhance your health. But it's good to know that if something unexpected happens to you, Ayurveda has your back. You will have access to an arsenal of Ayurvedic tools that are designed to empower you and give you your life back.

The idea is to look at the whole person in Ayurveda and to incorporate all the aspects of a person's life to help them restore their health. This includes learning physical exercises that stimulate health, knowledge of energy systems both within and outside the body and your own individual sense of being in the world. When you couple this with natural skin care, massage and regenerative remedies you will find that you have a treasure trove of Ayurvedic assets that will be there for you for many years to come. The case studies are rich and incredibly sophisticated. There will always be a chance to enhance your knowledge base. The world needs more practitioners and clinical professionals who can share in this knowledge. This will help us evolve, grow and set the stage for future generations.

CHAPTER 5

Exercise for Your Dosha

"If you would seek health, look first to the spine."
— Socrates (469-399 BC)

What kind of exercise do you do? If you are like most people, you may not be consistent with your current exercise routine. Exercising for your dosha type is based on integrating movements and routines into your current lifestyle that will create spinal flexibility. It's designed to boost your *prana* or energy by finding creative ways to use your spine. Modern exercise systems that are popular in gyms and sports clubs are limited in their planes of motion and tend to be much more linear in nature. The sketch below of Leonardo DaVinci's picture of Vitruvian Man illustrates the other planes of movement that the human body can move within. And if you really want to keep your spine strong and flexible, it is recommended to use a variety of movement directions. There are five possible movements of the spine: forward flexion (bending forward), lateral flexion (bending sideways), spinal extension (bending back), rotation (twisting movements) and circumduction (moving in a circle, although this is a move more common in the dance arts). To give you a hint on how to do spinal circumduction, you could move your spinal column in a circle, which is a little woozy or Sufi-dance feeling in nature.

Here is Da Vinci's Vitruvian Man:

This chart illustrates the multi-dimensionality of the human body. This is something that should be taught as part of everyday movement and exercise systems.

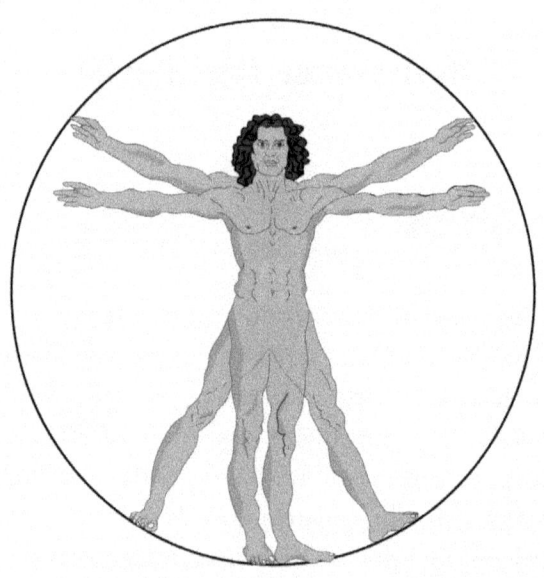

Multi-Dimensional Vitruvian Man

When you start embracing the concept of dimensions in movement patterns, your body's movement through space can be perceived more creatively. When some of these creative movement ideas are added to your everyday routine, like jogging, for example, you can tailor them to suit your body's constitution. Exercising for your dosha type can revitalize your energy levels. You will feel more alive and grounded. The types of exercises that I "prescribe" to clients include yoga-based postures, calisthenics, high and low intensity aerobic exercises, and stretching exercises. Yoga is a complete system of exercise and has been used for centuries in Ayurveda. Yoga exercise allows a complete range of motion for both the spine and the joints of the body. When you learn to exercise for your dosha, you will learn about some of the energy systems of the body that run through channels (called *nadis*) and how to activate them. These energy channels are involved in all bodily functions and can be activated by the positioning of your spine in conjunction with your breathing. The activation of these channels will increase blood flow and circulation in the body. It will also help remove toxins.

Have you ever left an exercise class or gym workout and felt tired? Have you ever felt like somehow you didn't burn calories, or you didn't feel great afterward? More than likely your energy was blocked from flowing at its best in your body. It could present itself as a blocked nerve, a tight muscle mass, a swelling or even a decrease in your range of motion. These things are very easy to monitor if you know what you are looking for. You can also change and heal them with energy point activation.

My client Erik is a dominantly *pitta* (fire) dosha constitution with some *vata* too (airy and scattered focus). Being the ambitious and determined *pitta* that he was, he was so busy working at his desk job that he decided to work out by carrying heavy bags on his commute every day. He was able to work his arms, and the weight-bearing exercise was good for bone density. But it was wrong for his dosha type because he had no stretching and spinal movements, which would have balanced out the loads he was carrying to work. He was also a chronic tooth grinder when he came to me and was clearly overworked and stressed. Erik was also taking heart medication for his blood pressure. He was a typical *pitta* in that he found it easy to lose weight and he had decent muscle mass, but he was becoming too skinny.

As we explored his dosha (dosha here meaning problem areas of the body) more in depth, I discovered adrenal stress indicators (*pitta* imbalance) and also that he needed to incorporate slower, more sustained movements into his workouts. He gets bored easily and it would take a lot of persuasion, but I was able to convince him to add deeper stretching and some soothing yoga poses into his manly routines. He made time to do this at night and sometimes on his lunch break. We kept it super simple and easy to execute. I taught him a slower version of the sun salutation series (*Surya Namaskar*) and we built momentum toward the last few rounds of the sun salutation series. Then I added other variations like the forward bending poses and some back extending poses. We would do a light spinal twist toward the end of the exercise routine. Since he was so pressed for time and I knew that he would not stick with it if it were longer, I kept the initial routine time at 40 minutes. He was eventually able to make more time to exercise, because he started feeling the health benefits sooner than he expected. He gradually quit drinking coffee and his bruxism (teetth grinding) finally disappeared over time. He became lighter on his feet and calmer.

There are lots of people like Erik who need help in slowing down their *pitta* constitution and who may be experiencing *pitta* imbalances. If left unattended, his bruxism would have gotten worse, and he could have fallen into a rut because he was not harnessing the right types of exercises for his constitution.

My client Scott was completely different. He was overweight and not as stressed about life as Erik was. He had *kapha* constitution and had become too comfortable eating and hardly exercising at all (*kapha* imbalance presents as excess amounts of the elements earth and water in the system). He needed to be up and moving because his doctor had diagnosed him as pre-diabetic. When he came to me, he had just started walking every other day and he was averaging a few thousand steps at first, which was nowhere near what he needed to do for his pre-diabetic situation. In addition to pre-diabetes, he had sinus issues that needed to be addressed. A sinus issue is a *kapha* issue too. Here it is indicated as a "*kapha* imbalance" when there is an "issue." It was clear he needed to get his heart rate up, so we built up speed on the treadmills with a gradual walk/light run combination and we made it easy to incorporate into his day. For Scott, work was his life. It was a sedentary work life, with a long commute as accounting manager for his office. Although there was pressure to perform in the office, his natural *kapha* (*kapha* as personality and physio type) nature allowed him to take the pressure in his own stride. But he needed to move, or he would be headed toward a more serious health situation down the road.

He started to take short breaks where he was able to add some light cardio exercises and stretches. After the first few weeks, he started noticing a boost in his energy from the spinal stretches and breathing exercises I had given him. He became motivated and started adding in a half-hour workout on the weekend days as well. We also integrated proper times of day for him to eat that worked best for his digestive *agni*. Very soon the pounds started coming off. He lost a total of 50 pounds over time and ended up leaving his job for one with shorter hours and demands. He is now putting together a wellness program in his current office where health professionals come in once a week to teach his co-workers how to maximize their wellness during lunch breaks. This was an unexpected surprise, and I was amazed at the initiative he was taking. I truly believe once a person starts noticing the health benefits of exercising in this way, they may want to show others how to do the same. Hey, if you don't intervene for someone you care about, who will?

Ayurveda embraces all exercise systems, but yoga poses are the most common recommendations for working out according to your dosha. These days there are many different types of yoga, but I recommend a knowledge of classical yoga poses for optimum health. A good yoga class will include a proper mix and timing of the twelve main yoga poses. The general actions that help create a healthy spine are flexion (forward bending), extension (back bending), lateral flexion (side-bending) and rotation (spinal twisting). These take place on one of three planes of motion.

PLANES OF MOVEMENT

Here are the planes of movement to consider.

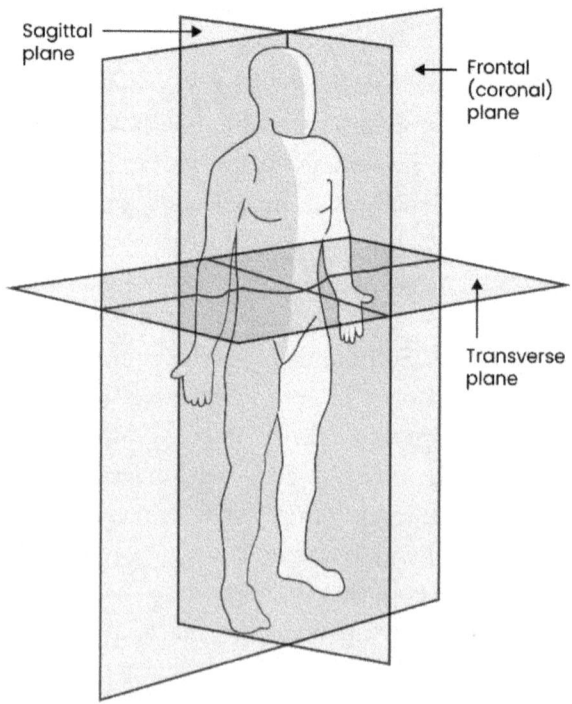

Here are twelve basic yoga poses that are beneficial to learn:

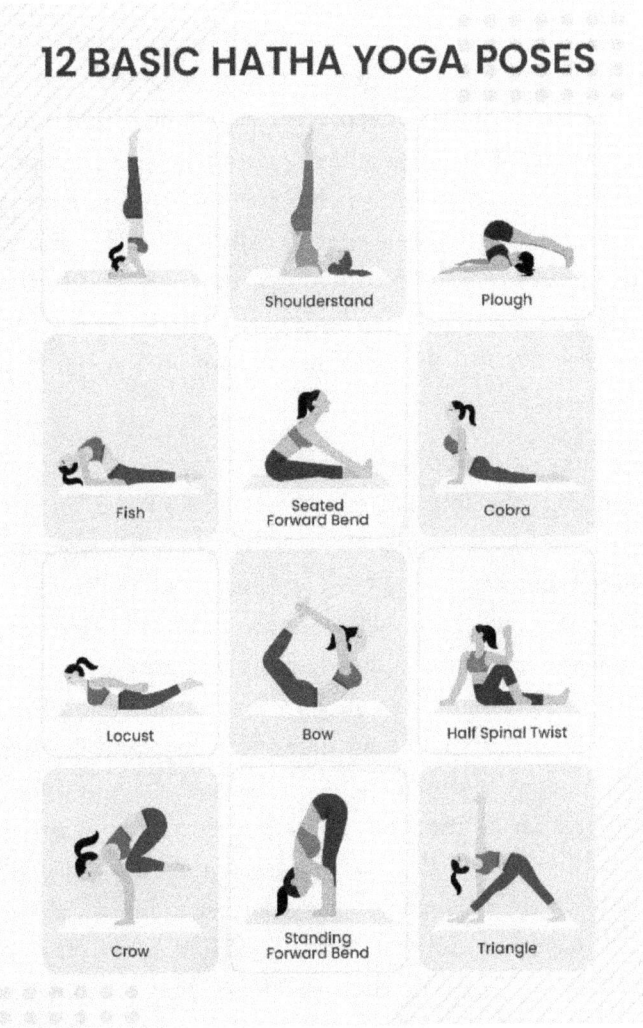

THE TWELVE ESSENTIAL YOGA POSES

Here we have a wide range of movement that is designed to relax and stimulate the energy systems in the body. The basic poses and stretches can be added to any busy schedule. You can shorten the yoga workout so that you do a little every day or every other day.

A mini yoga workout can be as short as 15 or 30 minutes. If you know what to do and are coached in how to start and finish, you will excel in this. You will find that just by being consistent, you'll be making progress. And, just like everything in Ayurveda, the benefits of the poses run deep. You will wonder why you didn't start this sooner. For those athletic types who feel yoga poses are about slowing down and not being fast enough, think twice. The building up of *prana* (internal energy) will be incredible and you will also be stimulating your digestive *agni* too. You will start feeling lighter and more connected to your body. This lends itself to more mindfulness in your daily life, You will be more present for others and for yourself.

When energy is blocked in the body from tight muscles or overexercising, the internal energy systems of the body cannot function at peak performance. The benefits of increasing your range of movement possibilities for spinal flexibility are incredible. Your neurological system will be more balanced. This will allow your brain and creativity to flow naturally. There are no benefits to be had from a stressful life and yoga poses will set you free. They will slow you down when your pressure is high and boost you up when your energy is low or stagnant. You can think of prana as the electrical system in the body. There are many energy pressure points on the body, called *marma points*, that we will explore in Chapter 9. There are many energy channels, or *nadis*, in the body in yoga. It has been said that there are 72,000 *nadis* in the body. In Chapter 6 we will explore the three main ones to know that will help you efficiently add breathing exercises to your everyday life. When focused breathing meets spinal flexibility, miracles happen. You can tap into energy fields on a subtle level if you understand this concept.

When my client Andrea came to me, she was suffering from anxiety and digestive issues. An Ayurvedic consultation revealed indicators of a fatty liver and the presence of *ama* or toxicity. She clearly wasn't digesting her food well and the more in-depth questioning revealed that she ate at erratic times and on the run literally. Andrea is an avid runner and was constantly suffering from some type of calf injury or foot problem. She was *vata* (air) dominant with *pitta* (fire). She was obsessed with running to "blow off stress" at work and she said she felt most free while running. She participated in half marathons and was athletic most of her life. This was all fine, but wear and tear at the joints and tendons was catching up to her along with repetitive stress. She needed to change her exercise routine to support her dosha. Her current pattern was burning her out: short warm-ups and not enough cool-down at the end of runs. Her poor calves didn't stand a chance and her digestive and stress issues just compounded the problem. I felt that we caught all this just in time. I started integrating a few spinal movements that she was not used to doing: spinal twists, forward bending exercises, and what I call a prescriptive "downward dog" series. For Andrea, the downward dog was such a relief for her calves and her back. It was also a chance to challenge herself by performing movements that provided relief from the repetitive stress of running. I showed her a simple downward dog routine and integrated exercise dyna-band stretches for her calves. As a result, she started feeling less tired after a few weeks of committing to this.

Because her stress levels were so high and because we treat the whole person in Ayurveda, I recommended some essential oils to be added to a nightly bath with Epsom salts. We integrated herbs and foods to boost digestion. She started switching out peppermint and chamomile tea for coffee and hot chocolate. She added fasting at nighttime and started taking holy basil (Tulsi) and dandelion. Andrea started to love the "work," as she said it was pleasurable, and she gradually loved the exercises once she saw how they were helping her.

The medical community has supported the benefits associated with yoga practice. They have taken note that with continued practice a person will notice a gradual loosening of the muscles and connective tissues that surround the bones and joints. This has supported the idea that yoga exercises contribute to reduced aches and pains. It can also help with other more serious conditions like arthritis, osteoporosis and back pain. It helps restore and preserve the cartilage surrounding the joints and bones by supplying fresh oxygen and blood to the area. It has been used extensively for people with disabilities and back pain. It has been shown to increase proprioception and an individual's ability to balance.

Yoga exercises can also be cardiovascular in nature when you take a series like the sun salutation and speed it up. There is no doubt that the increased oxygenation in the blood and the improved warming up of the circulatory system improves overall wellbeing while simultaneously allowing the body to rid itself of toxins. Those who practice yoga report improved digestion, calmer nerves and increased strength due to the time spent using your own body weight to increase resistance in the muscles. Many modern medical doctors have understood that yoga exercise can reduce the risk of heart attack by helping to thin the blood. The inversion exercises where you are balancing upside down contribute to increased circulation of stagnant blood in the body especially around the organs. It has also been beneficial for carpal tunnel syndrome and for people with injuries who are able to explore an increased range of motion by moving the body in different planes of motion. Essentially you are moving the spinal column and releasing tension in your neurology.

Yoga prescription exercises for a dosha imbalance are all part of a well-balanced health care protocol that supports the whole person. If the range of motion of a runner is increased in their joints and tendons they can run with more endurance with less risk of injury, This peace of mind will reduce their stress levels as they get to enjoy more of what they love. For the *kapha* person who needs to speed things up to burn fat, the exercises can be sped up, but they will also find benefits from a series that keeps moving and does not allow them to get "too comfortable." The beauty of increased spinal movements is that the endocrine and nervous systems will be stimulated to perform at their best.

I think you can see that the stage is set here for a long life if one were to start adding these empowering exercises to their Ayurvedic program. Energy is a precious commodity to waste, so if you feel something is missing in your current exercise routine, chances are something is missing. You will be able to fine-tune what is missing by incorporating balancing your dosha nature with an exercise routine that truly supports your energies and your personal quirks. Increased prana or vital energy will allow you to carry out your day with more power and grace. Of course, a key component in any exercise program is making sure you are breathing with maximum efficiency for the types of exercises that you are doing. Knowledge of pranayama or yogic breathing exercise can save you years of stress and worry and will improve your overall cognitive abilities by supplying more oxygen to both your body and your brain. Let's take a look!

CHAPTER 6

Breathing Exercises / Pranayama

"Remember to breathe. It is after all, the secret of life."
– Gregory Maguire, *A Lion Among Men*

Breath is the essence of life, and if harnessed properly, it can empower your soul. It can be used in Ayurveda as a recommendation to add to your daily routine. Breathing exercises or *pranayama* can be a powerful tool for your wellbeing and there are so many health benefits. The thing that appears to stop people from performing daily breathing exercises, or pranayama, is that it seems too complicated. Let's simplify the concept into two main things: 1) learn three basic pranayama exercises, and 2) practice them often. Repetition can allow them to become a habit. For beginners, breathing exercises are easier to do when you use shorter holding and releasing times.

Pranayama comes from the following words in Sanskrit:
Prana – "life force" or "life energy"

Yama – "discipline" or "control"
Ayama – "expansion," "non-restraint" or "extension"

Pranayama exercises are designed to cleanse and oxygenate the body and the mind. When you engage the nostrils in a pranayama exercise it can connect your conscious mind to your superconscious mind according to the yogis. Your breathing apparatus (diaphragm, mouth, lungs and nostrils) can be a superhighway to clarity of thought, calmness of spirit and increased oxygenation of the blood. Allergies and sinus problems are common ailments that can be healed by learning to use the micro and macro muscles that govern breathing. It's helpful to know the anatomy of the breathing apparatus in your body.

Let's look at the diaphragm:

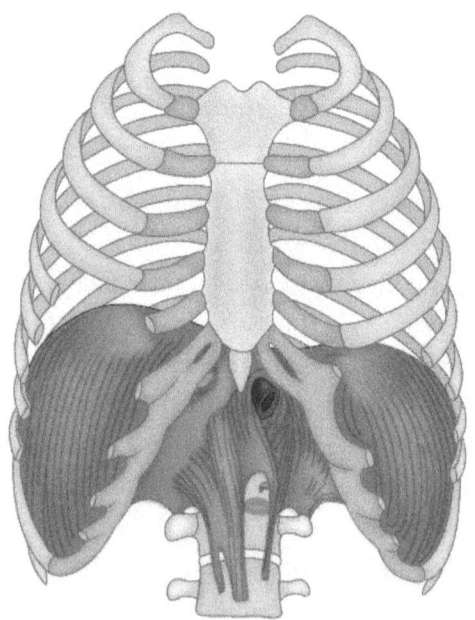

HUMAN DIAPHRAGM

The diaphragm functions like a balloon inside the body and attaches to some very important parts of the body: the lower ribs in front and thoracic vertebrae (T7-T12), and lumbar vertebrae (L1-L3) in the back. It also attaches to the *xiphoid process* or lower sternum in the front. Activating the diaphragm through pranayama exercises can help with lower back issues and with postural issues in the spine. The increased oxygenation of the blood and the resulting relaxation that occurs in your body is one of the main benefits that you will experience when you learn the biomechanics of pranayama. Once you understand the way the body works when you practice, you will be able to practice a little every day. These pranayama exercises can be used to release tension in the body, increase blood flow and clean toxins out. It is one of the cornerstones of yogic science. There are many types of breathing exercises that help with various energy systems in the body, and we will explore three of them in this chapter. We will also look at the basic types of breathing exercises that are beneficial for your dosha or personality/physio type. Please note that it is not essential to do a pranayama practice according to dosha, but knowing its effects on the body is a valuable tool for management of the doshas. The ultimate goal of pranayama is to calm the mind and prepare it for meditation. The three exercises we are going to discuss in this chapter are the bellows breathing, breath retention exercise and alternate nostril breathing.

The three breathing exercises and their Sanskrit names are:

Alternate Nostril Breathing *(Nadi Shodhana)*: connects two main nerve and subtle channels in the body called Ida and Pingala. The benefits are incredible. It involves breathing in through one nostril, retaining the breath with both nostrils and then exhaling through the opposite nostril. It alternates like an electric current from side to side.

Breath Retention *(Kumbhaka)*: this exercise oxygenates the blood and improves circulation. It can be performed after an exhalation, when the lungs are empty, or after an inhalation. I am choosing to teach this exercise with breath retention after inhalation. We are focusing here on *kumbhaka*, or holding of the breath after we inhale a breath.

Bellows breathing *(Bhastrika)*: This is a healing pranayama practice that involves filling and emptying the lungs and abdomen with air in a bellows-like fashion. It is performed gently yet powerfully by using your intention and your abdominal muscles. We never strain during these exercises, and we always allow the body to adjust naturally without forcing it. This eases the competitive brain during the process and allows you to "just be present" with the breath.

These three pranayama exercises can be practiced together, and if practiced often, you will find anxiety relief and a sense of calm that can be quite amazing. There are more breathing exercises in yoga as a person advances but these three are quite sufficient and have the qualities that will contribute to your health, wellbeing and calmness of mind for many years.

So let's explore some of the pranayama exercises. Alternate nostril breathing or *Nadi Shodhana* is a powerful balancing exercise for the sympathetic/parasympathetic nervous systems in the body. The research on the benefits of *Nadi Shodhana* is astounding. In Sanskrit, *nadi* means "channel," which refers to energy channels in the body; *shodhana* means "cleaning or purifying." So, *Nadi Shodhana* or alternate nostril breathing refers to the purifying of the energy channel by adding oxygen.

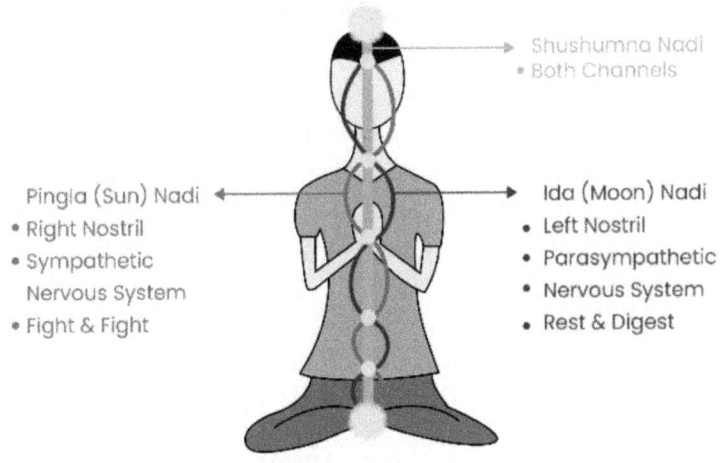

See the chart above.

NERVE ENERGY FLOW DURING ALTERNATE NOSTRIL BREATHING

Nadi Shodhana helps to balance the sympathetic "fight or flight" aspect of the peripheral nervous system, which is associated with the right nostril, with the parasympathetic nervous system, which is associated with the left nostril. These *nadis* or nerve channels are called *Ida* and *Pingala* and they crisscross internally in the body around *Sushumna nadi*, which is the subtle spine (meaning the spinal cord within the spinal column). It starts at the base of the skull and goes to the base of the spine. The three main subtle nerve channels that we focus on in this pranayama exercise are called *Sushumna*, *Ida* and *Pingala*. Knowledge of these energy centers can breathe life into yoga postures. You can consider these nerve channels as the body's electrical system. For more advanced yogis, it is along *Sushumna nadi* that the *Kundalini* energy gets awakened. These *nadis* channels are subtle and activated by the breath. For Ayurveda clients we recommend these exercises be incorporated into their daily lifestyle and routine choices. We recommend making it a simple habit instead of a chore. It's important to be gentle on yourself when you do it because the rewards of the practice will gradually become part of your psyche. These three exercises are the main ones that you really need to know for a healthy daily routine. For all the breathing exercises, sit in a comfortable cross-legged or seated position and wear loose-fitting clothing. Make sure you won't be disturbed. Remember, this is your time for your health. So, let's start.

PRANAYAMA EXERCISE 1: *NADI SHODHANA* (ALTERNATE NOSTRIL BREATHING)

Alternate Nostril Breathing / *Nadi Shodhana*:

This is an incredible exercise for awakening the prana or energy in the body. Clients report feeling more clarity of thought, and also feeling calmer, healthier and lighter after performing the exercise. It is considered a cleansing exercise because it helps cleanse the sinuses and strengthens the breathing apparatus in the body. When you start to practice alternate nostril breathing you can tap into your own creative potential and see where your breath flow may be blocked or where it may need some TLC. The simplest way to begin alternate nostril breathing is to start in a seated comfortable crossed-legged position. If it is uncomfortable for you to sit in that position, then sit in a chair.

You will be inhaling through one nostril, retaining the breath and then exhaling through the other nostril for a ratio of 2:8:4. The left nostril is the path of the *nadi* called Ida; the right nostril is that of Pingala. One round of *Nadi Shodhana* is made up of six steps. Start by practicing three rounds and then build up slowly to more.

Hand Position for *Nadi Shodhana*: This hand position is easy to do and is called "Vishnu Mudra."

Here is how it works: We are doing a ratio of 2:8:4 and we will be doing three rounds. You will notice a difference when you start doing a few rounds each day or every other day.

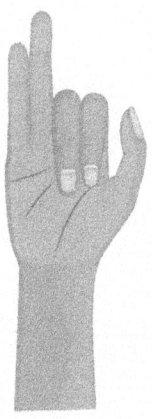

Start with your right hand in Vishnu mudra, which is pictured above. Use Vishnu *mudra* or a hand position where you start with your right hand and tuck your middle and index fingers in your palm and then raise your hand to your nose. Then you place your thumb by your right nostril and your ring and little fingers by your left.

1. Breathe into your left nostril for 2 counts while closing your right nostril with your thumb.
2. Hold your breath closing both nostrils and retain the breath for 8 counts.
3. Then breathe out through your right nostril, keeping your left nostril closed with your ring and pinky fingers for 4 counts.
4. Breathe in through your right nostril, keeping your left nostril closed for 2 counts.
5. Hold your breath closing both nostrils for 8 counts.
6. Breathe out through your left nostril, keeping the right closed with your thumb for 4 counts.

This is one round. Start your first time with three rounds and remember to go gently. This will grow on you, and you will find it is the simplest form of life insurance that you can get. Clients report feeling relaxed and calm, and others feel that it relieves anxiety and sinus problems. The exercise looks like this:

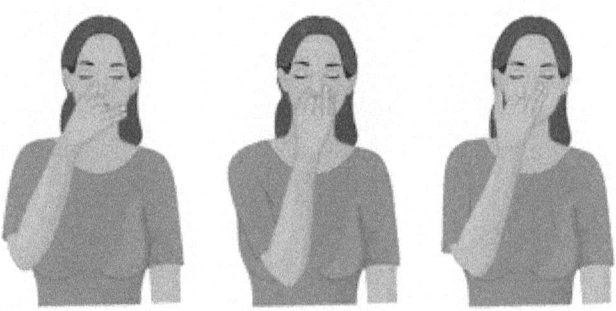

It can be performed for a few minutes in the morning or at the end of the evening. Just tailor it to your schedule and allow yourself to tune into the subtleties of the exercise. This is not a contest but a process that can help prepare your mind for meditation.

PRANAYAMA EXERCISE 2: *BHASTRIKA* (BELLOWS BREATHING)

Bhastrika in Sanskrit means "Bellows."

Repeat after me and say the command word "Ex-hale!" accenting the "Ex" in "Ex-hale!" Do this 10 times: "Ex-hale! Ex -hale! Ex-hale! Ex-hale! Ex-hale! Ex-hale! Ex-hale! Ex-hale! Ex-hale! Ex-hale!"

Great! Now repeat it again and this time use more energy. This time when you say the "Ex" syllable of the word "Exhale!" you contract your tummy in and exhale through your nostrils at a brisk tempo. Your body will naturally be sipping in little breaths in between exhalations. Picture your body like a bellows that is used to stoke a fire. Practice a few times, remembering you are no longer saying the word exhale, you are just silently performing the exercise to understand the mechanics. Once you feel you understand the coordination of the belly pushing in on the exhalations and the nostrils simultaneously exhaling, you have a bellows breathing happening. Congrats!

Now that you know the rhythm and you know that it will only be your tummy muscles and nostrils working, you will have good form for *Bhastrika*. Now that you understand biomechanics, let's do the actual exercise.

Sit in a comfortable, cross-legged or seated position and rest your hands on your knees. This exercise consists of a series of inhalations and exhalations where you are relaxing the shoulders but allowing your abdominal muscles to do the bellows action. Take two deep breaths, filling your belly with air. Keep your mouth closed and inhale and exhale rapidly through your nose while pulling your abdominals in on every exhalation like a pump. This will help to expel air from the lungs. Your inhalations and exhalations should be the same length and they are short. Start with a round of 10 and see the picture below:

Inhale a deep breath and exhale to prepare. Take another deep breath and begin.

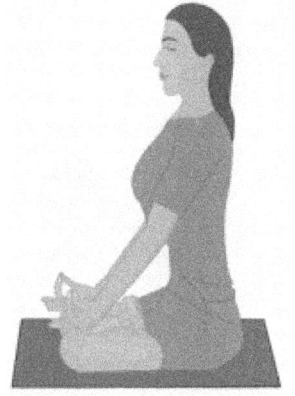 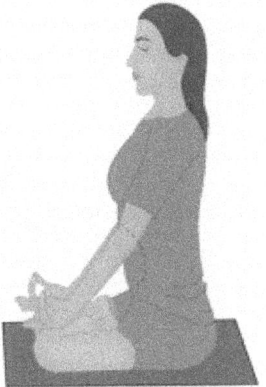

BHASTIKA BELLOWS BREATHING WITH ABDOMINAL CONTRACTIONS

Silently, just pushing the abs in and exhaling through both nostrils like a bellows. You've got this! "Ex-hale, ex-hale, ex-hale, ex-hale, ex-hale, ex-hale, ex-hale, ex-hale, ex-hale and then ex-hale one more time releasing all the breath. Relax. You can build up to 20 exhalations in no time once you understand the action the body takes in order to perform the bellows action.

PRANAYAMA EXERCISE 3: *KUMBHAKA* (BREATH RETENTION)

Kumbhaka means "pot" in Sanskrit (here it refers to the human torso as a pot with two openings)

There are many variations of this exercise but for simplicity's sake, we are just going to develop the endurance for retaining the breath after inhaling a deep breath. Basic breath retention or basic *kumbhaka* is all we need to know here.

Kumbhaka pranayama is another one of the traditional pranayama breathing exercises of Hatha Yoga.

Here are a few things to remember when performing this or any pranayama exercise:

- Don't hold your breath by force; don't go beyond your capacity as that defeats the purpose.
- Try to have an empty stomach before practicing.
- Also try to be in a relaxed state before performing this.
- Have a timer nearby.
- We will start with 30-second holding times and gradually and naturally increase from there.
- For everyday purposes of health and wellness you will usually build up to a minute or so of breath retention.

- Always practice sitting up in a cross-legged position or sitting in a chair.

I recommend touching your thumb and your forefinger together in a hand position or *mudra* called "chin mudra. This mudra symbolizes that "You and the Creator are One" and is a great hand position to get used to when you do *Bhastrika* pranayama.

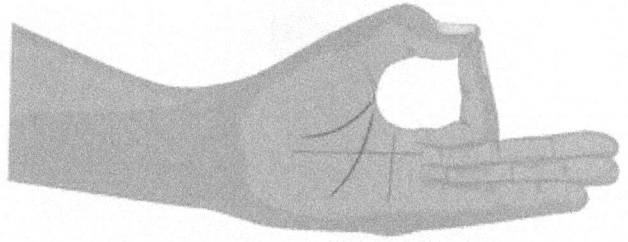

So, let's begin.

CHIN MUDRA

Sit in a comfortable position. Put your hands in chin mudra (touching the thumbs and the forefingers together).

Relax your eyes and the muscles around your jaw, shoulders and neck. Allow your back to be supported by your breathing. You can use pillows for support if you have back problems. Just focus on your breathing for a moment. Feel the breath come in through the nostrils and allow it to go out through the mouth. Have a phone timer or a stopwatch ready and set it for 30 seconds. Now inhale a deep natural breath through your nostrils and hold it for 30 seconds. Allow your body to be steady like a mountain. Notice the passage of time and when the timer buzzes gently release the breath through the mouth and relax. You can gradually increase your holding or retention time as you get better at this. If you allow your body to not resist and you focus on the miracle of the breath moving through your body, you will start to notice the health benefits.

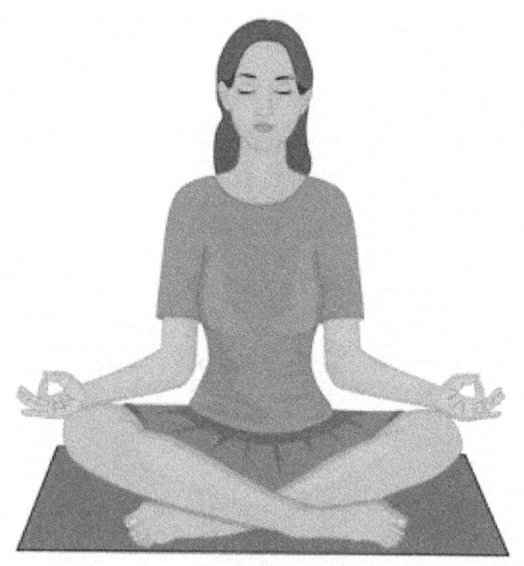

BREATH RETENTION EXERCISE

There you have it. Just learning these three exercises and practicing them a little every day will boost your health. There are many variations of pranayama exercises. I recommend keeping it simple by really learning and knowing these three exercises. You will have a lifetime of practice with these three gems. They will deepen any yoga practice and will aid athletic endurance in sports. They will prepare you for meditation or deepen your current meditative practice. Pranayama exercises can help already healthy people to become super-healthy. Research has illustrated the many health benefits, which include increased lung capacity, strengthening of the diaphragm and increased circulatory benefits. The *Bhastrika* bellows exercise has been said to improve the tone and functioning of internal organs, including the liver.

For Ayurvedic prescription pranayama, I may prescribe certain variations of these exercises to balance a person's dosha. Here dosha is used to denote imbalance within the body and not to describe your personality. So, if you are a *kapha/pitta* type with a *kapha* imbalance like being overweight or having an underactive thyroid, I might add more *Bhastrika* to your routine in order to enhance the other Ayurvedic remedies you are already doing. You can see how the bellows exercise would be very beneficial for the toning of the abdomen. Most obese individuals can't even feel their abdominal area and this exercise allows you to increase your body awareness and start to take control of toning and cleansing this area.

Over the years the clients who have been consistent with these exercises have all said that it supports their overall wellbeing. Health issues dominating our current world are mostly cardiovascular and toxin related at the cellular level. So much of the modern-day mental plight of obesity is emotionally rooted in incorrect ideas of helplessness, being too old, hormone imbalances and job stress. When you can calm yourself and purify your thoughts, you will find that balancing hormonal levels and weight loss become easier to achieve. You can start to come home to your innate state of homeostasis. Pranayama shows the way and is an integral part of any Ayurvedic protocol. Diet is the next frontier to explore, and Ayurveda has a lot to say about this. Let's go!

CHAPTER 7

Know Your Kitchen (Herbs, Spices and Plants)

"Food is our common ground, a universal experience."
– James Beard

In Ayurveda the kitchen has become a transformative place. You will be concocting easy to digest meals and restoring your health while having fun with the herbs and spices. The kitchen is where a lot of the creations will take place and it is important to have the tools of the trade ready. So, let's look around and see what we need.

The kitchen should be a clear space so you will need to let go of any clutter in this area. You want to set up a nice vibe or Feng Shui for this special place. In modern life, the kitchen can sometimes be in disarray and may even feel neglected. So, let's show your kitchen some love by keeping it clean and clutter free and decorated with excellent tools of trade. The setting up of the kitchen is a big part of clean eating and we are setting the stage for you to nourish yourself and your family. As you let go of old foods and old containers and jars, you will be creating the space for some of the new foods that you are introducing.

If you already have a clear space set up, let's do a container checklist. Make sure you have glass jars, closed containers and a label maker. You will need these for grains, legumes, herbs and some spices. Do a refrigerator and cabinet survey and let go of old foods that no longer support you. You will know which ones they are: foods high in gluten, sugars and chemicals. Just let them go. Clean out and make space for the new members of your food family in your cabinets and refrigerator as you integrate these new foods with your current food choices.

Ayurvedic foods are very appetizing, flavorful and aromatic. They are healing when served in an inspiring atmosphere. The cleansing of toxins and the electrochemical vitalizing of the body is the main objective. Ayurvedic cooking is both an art and a science. The idea is to consume food in adequate amounts and to have the right combinations of foods. Many diseases come about because of inadequate amounts of food that are prepared in the wrong way. So, you can think of food as medicine and the process of preparing it can be very enjoyable and rewarding. In Ayurveda foods are classified into three categories: *Sattvic* (pure in nature), *Rajasic* (spicy or hot) and *Tamasic* (heavy). These three qualities of s*attva*, *rajas* and *tamas* are also used in yogic science and Ayurveda to describe qualities in people, places and things.

Sattvic foods are considered the most beneficial to the body and are a high component of the yogic diet since they are pure and rich in *prana* or energy. This makes sense since the body can do more when you nourish it with water-rich, pure nutritious food in adequate amounts. We can learn a lot from the yogic diet, especially when it comes to quantity. The idea after each meal is to feel that the stomach is not completely full but that there is a third of the space left in the tummy. Ideally you should eat a third liquid at meals, a third solid foods and leave a third of your tummy empty. Then food becomes energy because you are not wasting energy digesting and absorbing "extra" food and the body can focus its extra energy for other things. A yogic diet ideally includes some *rajasic* (spicy) foods and maybe even a few *tamasic* (heavy) foods. This is part of the balance we want in our food choices.

Some examples of *sattvic* or high prana (energy) foods are:

Fruits: pomegranate, coconut, mango, peaches, pears and figs

Grains: all sprouted grains, amaranth, quinoa, rice and wheat

Vegetables: lettuce, sprouts, parsley, sweet potato, yellow squash, green leafy vegetables and okra

Beans: mung lentils, yellow lentils, lima and kidney

Dairy: organic yogurt and milks

Meat: none

Rajasic foods are spicy and are considered stimulating and tempting. They usually are enjoyable and fun but can be more difficult to digest. They can be energizing but of a different nature. The idea is to eat these in moderation because your digestive system will thank you.

Some examples of rajasic (hot, spicy, salty) foods are:

Fruit: apples, sour apples, bananas and guavas

Grains: buckwheat, millet, rye and teff

Vegetables: cauliflower, potato, broccoli, tamarind, nightshades and pickles

Beans: toor dal, adzuki and red lentils

Dairy: sour cream and some cheeses

Meat: chicken, fish and shrimp

Tamasic foods are heavy and can create a sense of lethargy in the body after eating. All processed foods and meats are included in this category because of the toll they take on the digestive process. If you overeat in this category it will show up somewhere in the body. Some examples of tamasic foods are:

Fruit: watermelon and plums

Grains: any processed flour of any grain, white flour of any kind

Vegetables: garlic, onion and mushrooms

Beans: urad dal, pinto, black and pink

Dairy: aged cheeses

Meat: beef, pork and lamb

It can be fun and easy to introduce Ayurvedic foods into your daily life. We want to add grains and legumes and make sure we are familiar with the variety that exists in these categories. We also want to eat lots of fruit and vegetables. Make sure there is a rainbow of colors in your salads. "Rainbow" refers to the variety and color of the fruits and vegetables that you are eating. It is better to eat the whole plant than to take supplemental fruit and veggie capsules and powders. You should buy organic, and it is best to have the whole food as nature intended. You will also become familiar with the variety of nuts that you can add to porridges and salads and see how easy it is to get balanced nutrition from proper food combining. You will become familiar with a variety of herbs and discover how they help the body heal naturally and gently. You will also learn about different oils for cooking and "popping" spices that you can easily add to any soup or grain dish. You will be engaging your five senses of sight, sound, touch, smell and taste in the process. The concept of engaging the senses to make something become "real" or a tangible part of your life is fun. You become engaged with cooking for health and you learn to have a steadfast appreciation for it.

So, let's explore more of these fascinating new ways to look at food preparation and dining.

In Ayurveda, foods are classified into the five following aspects:

- The six tastes
- Heating or cooling energy
- Post-digestion effect
- Special properties

In Sanskrit, the word for taste is *rasa*. It means essence or delight and is a pathway from the mouth to the brain. The essence of the taste of the food stimulates energy or *prana* in the body, which in turn stimulates the *agni* or digestive fire. There are six taste categories in Ayurveda which originated from the five elements. Remember the five elements in Ayurveda are earth, air, space, fire and water. The six tastes are:

- Sweet
- Salty
- Sour
- Pungent
- Bitter
- Astringent

The idea in Ayurvedic cooking is to have moderate amounts of each taste.

Energy, or *virya* in Sanskrit, refers to an energy in the body that activates taste. It is fascinating because taste can set off a plethora of images and ideas in the brain creating a sense-sation! Here we are looking to see if the taste has a heating or a cooling property. Each taste has its own energy, either heating or cooling, and it is good to be familiar with this.

The post-digestive effect refers to a taste you experience at the end of the digestive process. The taste will be different once the digestive juices or *agni* start breaking down the food and it passes in the alimentary canal. This type of physiological detail is what allows you to tune into which foods are helping you and your constitution and which ones are taking a toll on your health. This awareness occurs on a subtle or obvious level. An obvious level would be heartburn, for example, or GERD. A subtle awareness involves a connection with the body, mind and breath. You go within to see how these foods are nourishing you. It's pretty cool. If you feel uncomfortable or lethargic after eating, chances are you either ate the wrong foods or are not efficiently digesting the food you ate.

The special properties refers to the essence of the herbs you are using. This is the essence of the herb that involves knowing which part of the plant you are using and its nutritional value. You will understand as you explore Ayurvedic remedies how to activate the essence of the herb. This is a key component in herbology. With Ayurvedic knowledge of cooking and preparing meals, you can become an herbologist and an alchemist. Did you know there are many varieties of lentils that you can add to your cooking that all have different digestive properties? Urad dal, mung beans and so many other varieties create a unique classification of lentil technology. When you start adding different spices you will be creating a digestive support system that will help your body assimilate the food. When you have digestive support for your body, you won't need as much emotional support from outside. A nourished and balanced body translates to a nourished and balanced mind. We will explore digestion more in the next chapter.

If your kitchen is organized and you have all your ingredients ready, cooking an Ayurvedic meal can be very simple. Take kichari or vegetable and grain porridge for example. It takes about 15 minutes to prepare and about 20-25 minutes to cook. Let's do a quick checklist for your kitchen. You should have the following ingredients handy: basmati rice, split mung beans, quinoa, ghee, olive oil and spices. For spices, let's start with cumin, coriander, turmeric and ginger. Make sure your vegetables are farm fresh and have pre-made chutney and yogurt on hand. It is interesting to note that most store-bought yogurt has been pasteurized and the beneficial bacteria are added afterward. You may or may not be getting active cultures. The microbiome or gut health is very important in Ayurveda, and you could say that most disease starts here. The microbiome is a main focal point of many nutritional product companies, but they don't teach you how to grow your own with homemade yogurt. Your goal is to have your body producing these bacteria naturally and to have your body produce its own enzymes. You can still use prebiotics and probiotics, but just try to become more self-reliant. Your body will thank you.

Keep your beans and grains in glass jars for easy measuring. I am recommending split mung bean lentils to start out because they are the easiest to digest and they are balancing for all doshas. Here whole green mung beans have been split and the green skins have been removed. It provides protein to your diet and is also astringent in taste. Ayurveda has certainly perfected the art of the lentil and it is so helpful to get to know your lentil varieties so that you can creatively mix and match them in different recipes.

Now let's get into the grains and the grain family of choices. Whole grains are members of the grass, or Gramineae family, and produce a dry, one-seeded fruit. The fruit is commonly referred to as a kernel, grain or berry. There are eight grains that come from cereal grass: rice, corn, wheat, oats, rye, barley, millet and sorghum. There is also ancient wheat: spelt and kamut. Whole grains are composed of three layers, which include the germ, the endosperm and the bran. Knowing your grain anatomy will help you to become familiar with which parts nourish your body the best. The germ of the grain is the innermost part and contains vitamins E and K, minerals, essential oils and protein. The endosperm is the center starchy part of the grain and comprises about 80% of the kernel. The bran layer is the outer layer and consists of protein, fiber, minerals and B-complex vitamins. There are alternative grains that come from broadleaf plants and not grasses and include amaranth, buckwheat, flaxseed and quinoa. They are not technically grains and are sometimes referred to as pseudo-grains.

I am recommending that you start with adding quinoa and split-mung lentils to your grain cabinet. I am going to recommend adding basmati rice that you can easily store in one of your glass jars. This is to get you used to adding rice and lentils to meals and you can jazz them up with vegetables, spices and herbs as we go along. Let's talk about spices in Ayurvedic cooking.

Spices are an integral part of your new Ayurvedic kitchen. The exotic colors and the beautiful aroma of the spices will enhance any meal and you can play with these in the kitchen. Spices can easily elevate an ordinary dish like quinoa to a sublime feast for the eyes and the tummy. I usually recommend specific spices and herbs to clients in addition to grains and legumes, depending on what they have going on with their health. An Ayurvedic consultation will allow you to go deeper into dietary recommendations. Why not get a fresh head start in your own kitchen? I want you to keep things simple when you are starting out because this is a whole new world for most folks.

When it comes to spices just remember that a little goes a long way and to use them in moderation. Most spices release their flavors and aromas best when sautéed in ghee, so please have a jar of ghee on hand. Ghee is clarified butter, and it is a rich source of vitamins E, D and K. It is made from cow's milk butter, which is created with low heat until the water evaporates, leaving behind milk solids. Because it is created under 100-degree heat, it retains more nutrients than standard clarified butter. You can also cook spices with oil, and this will be a useful cooking technique that you can use a lot as an Ayurvedic chef. You will let the spices "pop" to release the aroma and can easily add them to any grain dish. You will need to store your spices in airtight containers away from heat and light. I ask that you start to think of herbs and spices as your newfound friends in the kitchen. If they are new to you then you want to get to know them like a newfound friend. Taking the time to "get to know" them will reap Ayurvedic knowledge rewards, which will result in glowing health.

Turmeric is a heating spice and contains curcumin and is a staple in Ayurvedic cooking. It is a powerful anti-inflammatory that is great for gut health. It can easily be added to just about any dish and is also an ingredient in "golden milk," a recipe that I will share in the next chapter. Cumin is a cooling spice and is an excellent antioxidant with a lot of versatility. Fennel is a cooling spice and can be used for teas and soups. Eating a few after a meal is also very beneficial. Carom seed (which is a fruit) and bishop's-weed are powerful anti-inflammatories that are used in *Ajwain* tea and can easily be added to any lentil dish. Mustard seed comes from the mustard plant and is a powerful anti-microbial that can be used to enhance any meal. It aids in digestion and contains sinigrin. Other great spices to have on hand are cinnamon, clove, cardamom, anise and ginger.

Vegetables offer a lot of options, and they may have edible leaves, roots, stems and seeds. Each group will offer something different to the diet, but overall, you want to use a combination of raw and cooked vegetables in your Ayurvedic meal planning. The roots of some vegetables are rich in Vitamin B and the leaves, fruits and stems can be great sources of vitamins, minerals, roughage and water. I recommend experimenting here with color for your vegetables and whipping up creative dishes with some of the spices mentioned above. Broccoli, cauliflower, yellow squash, cucumber, tomato, sweet potato and green leafy vegetables are all great to have on hand. Your only limit will be your imagination!

Fruits should be a part of any healthy Ayurvedic diet. Ideally, we want to have copious servings (up to five or more) of fruits and veggies every day. There may be ways of preparing these that you never thought of that will make them tasty and fun. The most popular fruits that are used in Ayurvedic cooking are apricots, apples, berries, cherries, papaya, pears, prunes, cranberries and grapefruit. These can be spiced up and heated with cinnamon and nutmeg and you can create so many different fruit dishes with them.

We also use a variety of nuts as well as honey, which opens up creative possibilities for everything from tea to dessert. Nuts are a great source of protein and also rich in phytonutrients and antioxidants. They contain both mono- and polyunsaturated fats that are great for heart health. They are also rich in arginine, which can improve blood vessel function. I am not going to be talking about chicken, fish or beef recipes at all, but I include them in my consultations with clients who eat them. You may find that you start feeling so good with the plant-based foods that you gradually ease out of eating the animal foods. The reward will be how your body feels and how much easier it is to have a strong and flexible body.

Never underestimate the power of a good honey. There are eight types of honey in Ayurveda, which are based on the type of bee that collects it. There are four main types that are used most commonly. The *pouttika* type of honey is collected by very large bees and is tingly, the *bhramara* type is collected by large bees and is sticky, *kshoudra* is collected by medium-sized bees and is cold and light by nature and *makshika* is collected by small bees. Makshika is considered the most medicinal. Who knew there could be so many sweet variations in honey!

In the next chapter we will explore some basic go-to recipes that will ease digestion and help you on the way to enjoying and creating your Ayurvedic kitchen.

CHAPTER 8

Foods that Boost Digestion

"Happiness for me is largely a matter of digestion."
– Lin Yutang

The process of digestion takes tremendous energy and is a miraculous achievement by the body. Proper digestion is a huge focal point in Ayurvedic cooking. Stoking the digestive fire, or *agni*, is very important for vitality and energy production. Good digestion boosts your prana and you will be able to do more in the world. The goal of Ayurvedic cooking is to facilitate digestion and absorption of nutrients and to balance the elimination process. When you think about it, this elaborate energy system starts with the mouth, the brain, and then the food passes through the esophagus to the stomach where powerful acidic digestive juices break down the nutrients. These nutrients then pass through the small and large intestines, where they can get absorbed into the bloodstream. It's important to have an alkaline body and a clean terrain within the blood and the cells.

It's important to know the best times of day to eat when your digestive juices may be running high. For most people it tends to be in the afternoon. This can make intermittent fasting easier because if you are fasting you can take the night off and give your organs of digestion a break. Ayurveda provides smoothie recipes and juice fast recipes that will make the journey of fasting easier. Detox ghee is a great thing to have on a fast because anything introduced into a fasting body will be absorbed faster.

I am going to share some simple easy to prepare recipes that will give you a broad overview of the versatility of ways that you can integrate Ayurvedic meals into your current routine. Once you see how easy it is, you can get creative and have fun while boosting your digestive *agni*.

Now that you have your kitchen set up and are ready to start this journey, let's look at some of the Ayurvedic foods that will boost your digestion. The more you become familiar with the plants, herbs and spices that facilitate your digestion, the more Ayurvedic knowledge you will want. This is a good habit to get into. You may be surprised which plant foods, herbs and spices actually aid digestion. So, let's explore.

There is a one-pot porridge dish called kichari that is easy to make and is great for digestion. It consists of legumes (usually split mung beans), rice (usually basmati) or another cleansing grain, cleansing vegetables, herbs, spices, seeds and nuts. You can vary the ingredients to make it an interesting addition to any household meal, or take it alone. It is typically consumed at midday, but you can partake for breakfast or dinner too. It is a regular dish at yoga centers, and you can even buy it pre-made. Let's look at a simple kichari recipe that takes 15 minutes to prepare and that cooks for about 25-30 minutes:

Ayurvedic Porridge (Kichari):

Serves 2

Large stainless steel cooking pot

Bowls for the ingredients

1 cup split organic mung beans

½ cup basmati rice or buckwheat

5 cups water

3 teaspoons turmeric

4 teaspoons olive oil

7-8 stems basil, cilantro or other spices (nutmeg, cardamom, curry, cinnamon)

2 cups cleansing vegetables (broccoli, cabbage, Brussels sprouts, carrots, bok choy, kale or celery: you choose, and you can experiment)

4 tablespoons raw unsalted nuts of your choice (walnuts, almonds, cashews or pine nuts)

2 tablespoons raw unsalted seeds (chia, pumpkin, sunflower, sesame, flaxseed)

Pinch of salt (Himalayan salt preferred because of trace mineral content)

Rinse the rice and the beans. In a large pot, combine the water, beans and rice and bring to a boil. Reduce the heat to a low boil and continue the cooking for 25-35 minutes. Then add the olive oil, turmeric and Himalayan salt while cooking. It's important to keep stirring and you can add more water if necessary. Toward the end of the cooking, you can add the basil, vegetables, seeds and nuts. Serve with a fresh salad.

When you start experimenting with more bean types and longer cooking times you may wish to consider buying an electric pressure cooker. Ayurvedic chefs use an electric pressure cooker, which takes away the fear of having a lid explode. The beauty of this is you let the Ayurvedic casserole dish with all its wonderful healthy ingredients sit overnight and have a fresh meal in the morning.

Ayurvedic Fruit Stew

Serves 2

Ingredients:

½ cup dried apricots soaked at least 4 hours in filtered water

½ cup dried figs soaked at least 4 hours in filtered water

½ cup diced apple (preferably sweet)

½ teaspoon grated fresh ginger

½ teaspoon cinnamon

½ teaspoon nutmeg

A pinch of salt

2 teaspoons ghee

Filtered water as needed

Melt the ghee in a small pan and simmer the ginger, cinnamon and nutmeg until you sense the aroma is present. Add in the apple, apricots and figs with water that the figs and apricots were soaking in and start stirring the pot with the ghee and spice oil. Then add the filtered water to cover the fruit, cover and simmer until the fruit is tender (about 10 minutes). Turn off the heat and let the mixture cool for 5 minutes.

This is a great meal for digestive fire and is very filling and satisfying. You can modify the apple choice to more tart for a *kapha* dosha or mildly sweet like Granny Smith for *pitta* dosha. The sweeter apple type is generally good for *vata* dosha. Dried fruit is a great option in this recipe when you don't have a large variety of local fruits. Your digestive *agni* will be boosted by the reconstitution of the dried fruits with soaking for the 4 hours. This is the key to easy to digest food that is highly nutritious.

Ayurvedic cooking always emphasizes seasonal, organic and locally grown foods when possible. So have fun with this recipe during the seasonal changes with your newfound Ayurvedic knowledge.

Ayurvedic cooking involves engagement of all five senses as much as possible. Touching, seeing, hearing, smelling and tasting the food are all an integral part of the process. I remember when I first started doing this at home, my dog and my friends were captivated by the sensual process of Ayurvedic cooking. My dog almost became a vegetarian through this exposure (only kidding). The idea is to learn your different plant and legume varieties so that you can have versatility in your meal preparation. These foods will enhance your digestive *agni* while creating an inviting family atmosphere.

In Ayurvedic cooking there are six tastes as we mentioned earlier:

- Sweet (Madura) which consists of Earth and Water elements
- Sour (Amla) Earth and Fire
- Salty (Lavana) Fire and Water
- Pungent (Katu) Fire and Air
- Bitter (Tikta) Air and Space
- Astringent (Kasaya) Air and Earth

The word for taste in Sanskrit is *rasa*. The tastes that are included in the meals are designed to have a balancing effect on the doshas. Sweet taste in general is more grounding, sour is more appetite stimulating, salt is more electrolyte balancing and bitter taste is more cooling and detoxifying. The pungent taste is stimulating and is good for metabolism and includes foods like ginger, garlic and chili peppers. The astringent taste has a good drying effect in the body, helping to control excess moisture, and includes foods like legumes, green teas, and pomegranates.

Here is a nice chutney recipe that you can vary according to which tastes you want to add to your meal:

Tomatillo and Kiwi Chutney

4 Servings

Ingredients:

4 kiwis cubed and peeled

4 chopped small tomatillos

2 tsp lime juice

2 chopped green apples

2 chopped green chilis

½ cup fresh mint

½ cup chopped coriander leaves

½ cup grated ginger

½ tsp Himalayan salt

2 tsp roasted cumin seeds

Add all ingredients in a blender and put on pulse 4-5 times. Remove and store in a glass jar and refrigerate.

Just keep in mind that the Ayurvedic dietary protocol will never be strict (unless a person has a chronic or very serious health problem) and that there is flexibility within the system. Ayurvedic experts like to work with the client's existing diet so we will normally not ask you to quit chicken, fish or turkey if that is in your diet. The idea is to wean away from the heavier foods that will take more of a toll on your digestive *agni* and to move in the direction of a healthier balanced diet that has you feeling great in your skin. The only way to get there sometimes is to make it easily accessible and simple. Start adding some simple grain, soup, veggie, smoothie and fruit recipes to your existing routine and you will reap health benefits that are priceless. So, let's explore some common food products.

Milk is the only animal product that the animal gives willingly, and its benefits are wide in scope. It can be a rich source of calcium and vitamin D, but you want to keep it organic and chemical free whenever you can. You can easily make your own homemade milks from nuts (like almond milk, cashew milk and oat milk) and these are wonderful for digestion and all consistent with an Ayurvedic protocol. Sometimes when you buy store-bought nut milks there can be additives that you really don't want in your system. In order for the nut milks to last long in the grocery store they add these chemicals, and they can consist of acidity regulators like potassium hydroxide and tocopherols (Vitamin E) to retard spoilage. To maintain a consistent texture, emulsifiers and stabilizers like carrageenan are usually added. Why not just make your own? It's so easy to make your own nut milk. Here is one of my favorite recipes:

Homemade Almond Milk

3-4 servings

Filtered Water (start with one cup at a time to taste)

Handful of soaked raw almonds (organic, soaked overnight in enough filtered water to cover them)

1 tsp vanilla

¼ cup maple syrup (organic)

¼ teaspoon cinnamon

¼ teaspoon nutmeg

Ice (one or two cups made with filtered water)

Here it is beneficial to have a high-powered blender like a Vitamix blender. You want a high-powered blender with durable construction from a trusted name that will keep the whole food intact. Put the soaked almonds and their water in the blender. Add a cup of filtered water and blend so that the almonds are pureed. Add cinnamon, nutmeg, maple syrup and vanilla and a little more water. Blend this mixture another 30 seconds or so at a medium speed so that the mixture is well blended. Then add a cup of filtered ice and a half to a full cup of water to increase volume and blend again for another 30-45 seconds. Don't worry about a froth that appears, or a separation; that will depend on the almonds that you use. You can drink this plain or add organic cereal like steel-cut oats or granola. Pour any remaining mixture into a container and chill to have as a drink later. This almond milk recipe is best if consumed within two days. The idea is to make it fresh, and you will have delicious chemical-free nut milk.

Yogurt with beneficial bacteria intact is a great food for optimum digestive and gut health. It is best to make your own, but if you can't, try to find organic yogurt with active cultures. The cultures in a good store-bought yogurt will have the beneficial bacteria added after the pasteurization process. But let's see how easy it is to make your own. You can buy an automatic yogurt maker, but you will find it is easy to make your own.

Homemade Yogurt Recipe

Ingredients:

1 quart organic whole milk

2 tablespoons organic yogurt

Heat milk until foam appears. Turn off the heat and allow it to cool to about body temperature or about 100 degrees. You can use a food thermometer. Pour the milk into a sterilized glass jar. Mix in the yogurt, making sure it is at room temperature. Cover the jar with a lid and put in a warm place where there is no draft. Put it away for the evening and in the morning, you will have fresh yogurt with active cultures. Now let's try an Ayurvedic favorite yogurt drink, lassi. Lassi has many health benefits, as you can imagine.

Ayurvedic Yogurt Drink (Lassi)

Ingredients:

1 cup plain yogurt (homemade or organic)

¾ cup filtered water

¼ teaspoon cardamom powder

1 tablespoon honey

pinch of ground ginger

Combine the water, honey, yogurt, cardamom and ginger in a blender. Blend until the mixture becomes a little frothy and smooth. You can adjust the sweetness with the honey. Pour the lassi into serving glasses and serve chilled. Now let's try a variation of this theme.

Golden Milk Recipe

Ingredients:

1 cup milk (organic and can use coconut or almond milk)

2 teaspoons maple syrup or honey

½ teaspoon ground turmeric

¼ teaspoon ground cinnamon

A pinch of black pepper

Combine the milk, turmeric, cinnamon and pepper in a saucepan. Warm over medium heat, stirring often to prevent sticking. Heat until hot but not boiling. Remove from heat and let cool slightly. Stir in maple syrup or honey to taste. The turmeric makes the milk a golden color and is a powerful antioxidant. This is a nice drink with many health benefits that helps digestion and can be a great nighttime drink.

There are so many ways to boost digestion when you are dialed in to how the body and the mind work together. Intermittent fasting is a great routine to get into. You should base the timing on when you feel your body may have the most difficulty in digesting foods. For many people, this is in the evening hours, so a fasting period of say 8-10 hours from evening until morning (say starting at 7 p.m.) might work best. You can also do a one-day fast once a week for 24 hours. It may seem challenging, but it can give rise to a boost in food consciousness and clarity of thought, while giving your digestive organs a chance to chill and relax. This in turn will be very beneficial for that detox machine that is your poor liver. I know many of my dancer and performing artist clients swear by the one-day fast as they feel it helps them to maintain a more peak performance state in the days following and it helps to balance their weight. I add a little "fasting boost" smoothie to the one-day fast for my clients and it consists of detox ghee, avocado and broccoli, blended. Here is a recipe for the detox ghee that you can add to a fasting smoothie:

Detox Ghee:

1 lb unsalted butter

¼ cup chopped mint

¼ cup chopped coriander leaves

1/8 cup grated ginger

½ tbsp dry fenugreek leaves or ½ tsp triphala powder

Blend together the mint, coriander, grated ginger and fenugreek with some water to a fine paste. Then add the paste to the butter and heat on slow fire, stirring until granulated. Strain with a cheesecloth and store in a glass jar.

Triphala powder is a nice option in the recipe because it contains three dried fruits that are highly beneficial for digestion:

- *Amla* (Emblica officinalis): Indian gooseberry; digestive and immune system enhancer
- *Bhibhitaki* (Terminalia bellirica): great for respiratory system and general detoxification
- *Haritaki* (Terminalia chebula): excellent for elimination and has many digestive system boosting properties

Triphala has been used for centuries in Ayurveda.

As noted earlier in the book, ghee, or clarified butter, is another potent food used in Ayurvedic cooking and meal preparation. It is made by melting down butter enough to separate the milk solids, just leaving the butterfat, which is rich in omega-3 and omega-9 fatty acids as well as vitamins, K, D, A and E. It is considered a sattvic or pure food in Ayurvedic cooking. It is used as a carrier for Ayurvedic spices and herbs in many varied preparations. So, let's create a fasting one-day smoothie with detox ghee and either the fenugreek or the triphala. It's such a simple recipe and I would take it midway through a 24-hour fast along with filtered water. Of course, you don't have to be fasting to try it, but why not?

Fasting Smoothie

1 cup organic broccoli (kale can be substituted or a comparable green vegetable)

1 cup avocado

1 tbsp detox ghee

¼ cup filtered water

Blend all ingredients together on low-medium speed with water until smooth. Pour and serve. Congratulate yourself on a day well fasted.

I think you can see how the foods that benefit digestion are easy to prepare and add to any meal. You can play with ingredients and start to have an intuitive sense of which tastes and ingredients are beneficial for your dosha. Once you have an Ayurvedic consultation and tune into what areas of your body may be giving a subtle (or screaming) cry for help, you will be in a good position to start supporting the system that needs help.

It will be good to tune into the times of the day when you know your digestive fire or *agni* is naturally high and work off that. Giving your digestion a break in the form of mini-fasting breaks and intermittent fasting will be a huge system boost. When you think about what we put into our body over the period of the past few years, we can appreciate the amount of work it does to keep us healthy, wealthy and wise. Ayurveda shows the way and is all part of a lifestyle routine that can always be your true north. It will always guide you to health and boost your awareness to the point where you will be the healthiest person in a social setting, making naturally wise choices that boost your energy. Now let's explore an important part of the daily routine: setting up for sleep and yoga nidra.

CHAPTER 9

Yoga Nidra / The Five Sheaths

*"There is a time for many words and there
is also a time for sleep."*
– Homer

These days we need all the help we can get to decompress from the day's activities. Many people have trouble dozing off into a peaceful night's sleep. There is so much happening in modern life and many times sleep is neglected. There is conflicting info on how many hours of sleep a person should get, but one thing is certain: if you are able to decompress from the day and drift into a deep restorative sleep, the quality of sleep will be more important than the quantity. It's true that if you have been sleep deprived because of a hectic lifestyle and responsibilities, then you may need to give your body the benefit of longer hours of sleep at different times. Depriving oneself of sleep can contribute to adrenal stress and can disrupt the body's natural hormonal balance.

Ayurvedic recommendations are to fall asleep when you are naturally tired in an environment that is conducive to sleep. The idea is not to depend on any unnatural substances like sleeping pills or alcohol but to set a stage or ritual that will lend itself to a peaceful night's sleep. It is recommended to turn all electronics off and to have the environment be dark. Sleeping in the dark is part of a natural rhythm of sleep that depends on the natural daylight and nighttime. Of course, this could get confusing when you are traveling in different time zones or living in a country like Norway or Alaska where there are times of the year that consist of constant daylight or nighttime. Here you would need to adjust to a healthy rhythm of sleep based on what allows your body to function at its best.

I have a client who used to live in Norway, and he said the long winters were a depressing time and that this constant darkness made it easy to rely on escapist drugs or alcohol in order to offset the constant darkness. The best I can say here regarding environments like this is to change your lifestyle so that you are eating even healthier according to dosha and exercising even more according to dosha. Alcohol in this context is like putting kerosene on a fire to put it out. It will catch up to you in a short time and will take a toll on your liver and pancreatic health. Ayurvedic recommendations regarding alcohol are not to drink. I had an Ayurvedic physician and mentor who said that Ayurveda would be okay with drinking. The amount would be no more than a thimble full of an alcoholic beverage daily. This is amusing and also sad because it shows that there is no nutritional value in alcohol and absolutely no health benefit.

I know many client performers who have relied on alcohol for creativity or to loosen up their muscles for dancing or to help them sleep. I have weaned them off of this habit and started to see the dark circles retreat from their eyes in a short period of time. Also, they did not like giving up this habit so there was some resentment and also reliance on stimulants to offset the alcohol. When you are trying to cut down on alcohol, it is highly recommended not to rely on coffee or another stimulant to compensate. That won't bring nutritional and energetic balance. It can burn you out if you do not try to control it. Coffee in moderation, not compensation, should be the motto.

Just as the doshas of *pitta*, *kapha* and *vata* have a quality that describes personality and constitution, they can also be used to describe certain times of day:

Kapha time: 6a.m.-10a.m. and 6p.m.-10p.m. This a time for calmness and balancing in general, which is a *kapha* quality. *Kapha* is also associated with springtime and adolescence.

Pitta time: 10a.m.-2p.m. and 10p.m.-2a.m. This is a time for peak mental and physical activity. *Pitta* is also associated with summer and the prime of one's life.

Vata time: 2p.m.-6p.m. and 2a.m. to 6a.m. This time is for increased creativity and restlessness. *Vata* is wintertime and middle age and above.

So, what is the best time to decompress in Ayurveda? Ideally it is *kapha* time, when possible; physiologically speaking, it is a great time for the body's natural hormonal rhythm. Not everyone has the luxury of being able to sleep at 10 p.m. but maybe by 11 p.m. or later will still be a good option for replenishing the hormones. As you are creating this healthy lifestyle, you will be digesting your food better, possibly even fasting or semi-fasting at night, and you will be exercising in a manner that supports your energy. All these contributing factors will support a good night's sleep. You will sleep sounder when your tummy is empty.

As you explore the breathing exercises or pranayama, you are creating a meditative environment to allow your mind to relax and let go. Stress and anxiety will naturally release when you are feeling grounded and focused on your health. It's best to take it further so that you increase the chances that you will be receiving restorative, deep, regenerative sleep. Ayurvedic recommendations are to set up a sleep ritual that includes essential oils, hot baths, electronics off, and an environment that lends itself naturally to good sleep. I have clients complaining that they never have time to sleep at a decent hour because their minds are racing, or the kids are keeping them up. Whatever it is, allow whatever is getting in the way to change and create a "sacred space" around sleeping. The deeper you can sink into a good night's rest, the more creative energy you will have and ultimately the less sleep you will need.

This natural cadence of a sleep rhythm and a lifestyle that is conducive to deeper sleeping will allow you to use those hours for body and mind restoration and rejuvenation. You have a golden opportunity to support your self-care in the later evening hours, and Ayurveda has a plan that will support you. Let's start with a natural decompressing ritual that can support deep sleep. Couples need to understand each other's night rhythms and to allow them to come into sync with each other. There are herbs that support healthy sexual health and fertility in the context of healthy lifestyle in Ayurveda:

- *Shatavari* (Asparagus racemosus): This is considered a rejuvenating adaptogenic herb that is beneficial for female libido.
- *Ashwagandha* (Withania somnifera): This herb has many benefits, including boosting libido and reducing anxiety.
- *Safed Musli* (Chlorophytum borivilianum): This herb has aphrodisiac qualities and is beneficial for both men and women.

These natural enhancers should be considered under the recommendations of an Ayurvedic expert, and you should let your own primary care physician know so that you can make sure they don't interfere with any current medication. The idea is that you will already be feeling healthier by tuning into your body and your digestion, and there will be a lot of natural energy that you are producing, so your sexual prana will already be higher. It's amazing what you can do on your own to boost your health. A healthy sex life can allow you to drift into a good night's sleep and, when you are able to sync your sleep patterns with your partner's patterns, you will have more energy during the daylight hours too.

Nighttime can become a sensual ritual that supports a modern healthy lifestyle regardless of how much time you must put into it. Choose colors for your bedroom that are soothing and relaxing and use natural fabrics for your sheets, pillows and blankets whenever possible. Natural cottons and linens support a healthy sleep. There are so many styles of beds, but you want a mattress that supports your spinal health and natural sleep patterns. It should be a strong natural and flexible material. Taking a hot bath with Epsom salts and apple cider vinegar can relieve sore or tired muscles and boost magnesium in the body. Many professional dancers know this hack and it works like a charm. Just pour one cup of Epsom salts and one cup apple cider vinegar into a hot bath. Soak for half an hour, rinse off, and then prepare for sleep.

Nighttime is a great time to restore your hormones naturally. Cortisol is secreted by the adrenal glands that are on top of each kidney. Growth hormones (somatotropin or HGH) are secreted by the anterior pituitary gland. Melatonin, the sleep hormone, occurs naturally in darkness so that is why it is important to have lights out and electronics off as you prepare to retire for the evening. It is produced in the pineal gland. These glands and other glands, including the hypothalamus, the thyroid, the pancreas, etc., are all part of the endocrine system. Yoga exercises are the main exercises that stimulate the endocrine system by the positioning of the spine. As you integrate some of these spinal exercises into your daily routine, you will naturally be relaxing your nervous system and stimulating these glands to do their job. This all contributes to having a restful and restorative night's sleep.

Essential oils can play a role in deeply relaxing the nervous and limbic systems and allowing the body and mind to calm together to fall asleep. Lavender is deeply relaxing and can be added to the bath or a hot tea made with lavender flowers before bedtime. Each essential oil offers something different for everyone, so I recommend that you find an essential oil that you resonate with and use that. Rose oil is very soothing and blends nicely with lavender. It can be placed on the body (just a few drops on the wrists or the back of the neck) or it can be inhaled in a diffuser or another very simple method. Once you have tested the essential oil and know that you are not allergic to it, you can use this very simple aromatherapeutic procedure. I have used lavender in this example, but you can use citrus essential oils, peppermint or any others that are good for the respiratory system.

Take 3-6 drops of lavender in the palm of one hand. Take the second and third fingers of your opposite hand and swirl the essential oil in your palm in a circular movement for five or six swirls. Rub your two palms together a few times and then cup your hands around your nose and mouth without touching the skin on your face. Inhale the lavender oil through your nostrils for four counts and exhale naturally through your mouth for four counts. Repeat for five or six rounds. This mixture will start to relax your mind and will put your limbic system at ease. I have used this a lot with corporate wellness clients, and it can be used on breaks in the office. This will help you to feel more relaxed when you return to your cubicle. This technique can also be an excellent part of any sleep ritual. Some other essential oils that are conducive to sleeping include valerian, bergamot and frankincense. Have fun with these as you create your own sleep ritual that works best for you and your environment. Consult with an Ayurvedic expert when you want more fine tuning with essential oil selection, teas and herbs to help your dosha.

Yoga nidra is a great adjunct to any end of night routine and can be considered a guided mental imagery experience that is done while you are lying down in shavasana, or a corpse pose. It is guided to allow you to tune into your body and your surroundings in a deep way. It was introduced in the 1960s to the public through the writings of Swami Satyananda Saraswati. The goal of yoga nidra, or "yogic sleep," is complete relaxation. It is being practiced in many yoga centers and many practitioners claim that it is an effective stress management tool that helps you to actualize transformational goals. Clinical research has shown that yoga nidra has been associated with improved red blood cell counts, hormonal changes and blood glucose levels. Its effect on the central nervous system, or CNS, is measurable. There have been reports through two neuro-imaging studies that yoga nidra practice produces changes in dopamine release and cerebral blood flow.

I recommend taking classes in yoga nidra by a highly qualified teacher with whom you feel comfortable. You will find yourself practicing on your own at night as part of a decompressing ritual that is refreshing and enlightening. I do it often at the end of a long day in shavasana right on my bed, which is underneath a wonderful skylight. My home environment is set up where my bedroom is very quiet and conducive to relaxation. It is not too "busy" in terms of anything related to office or work. I have nothing like that in my room and it is very minimalist. This creates a sanctuary-style environment that allows me to feel totally at peace here. In learning and practicing yoga nidra, your connection with your environment will never be lost. The hyper-stimulating effects of your daily life are let go of and you become aware of your body in time and space. This allows you to change your perceptual perspective and open your mind to receiving transformational suggestions that are healing and uplifting in nature. This can become a deeper experience the more you practice it and can be perfumed during different times of the day as well. It has been said that during the deep state of relaxation that yoga nidra produces, an awareness of one's surroundings is increased and learning abilities are enhanced. This is a great way to disconnect from the overstimulating effects of your environment and move into a dream-like state.

Yoga nidra is practiced for about 30 minutes to an hour. When you are in the deepest part of the state here, practitioners feel that they are realigned with the most spiritual part of their inner nature. It is never a substitute for sleep, but the benefits will go far beyond it. It can be an integral part of any pre-sleep routine where you are setting up your space for the art of sleeping. One technique is learning to direct the focus on various parts of the body and allowing that part to feel tension and then to release the tension and let it go. You become an observer of your body here, and as you tense the area you bring awareness of what tension is and then let it go. Your senses will heighten, and the idea is to focus on the nowness of the moment. There are many stages of the yoga nidra process, so I invite you to explore them often. You are transforming your neurology to support your health and you will start to discover new ideas and thoughts when you allow the body to relax this deeply. It will support your health profoundly when you allow yourself to let go during this process.

When practicing yoga nidra, it will help to know the sheaths of existence which are called *koshas*. There are five sheaths, or *koshas*, that are thought to encase the soul, or Atman. You can tune into your soul nature according to this concept of the sheaths from the

Vedas. Some systems describe more than five sheaths, but we will focus on five sheaths here. See the chart below:

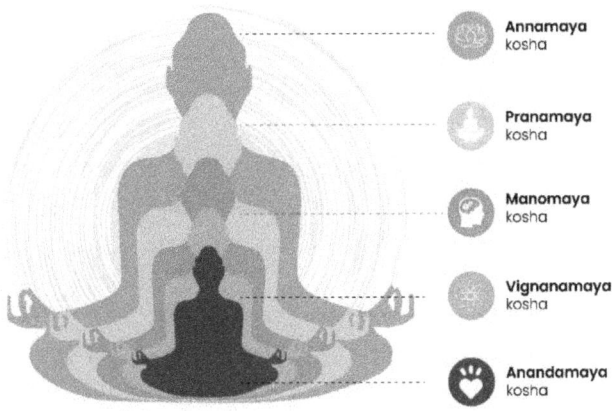

The Five Sheaths or Koshas:

- *Annamaya Kosha*: the physical body; made up of our muscles, organs, bones and matter. This is the most common layer of self that we are in touch with. Everything that we can experience through the five senses.
- *Pranamaya Kosha*: this is our energy body, including the body and the breath. It is also considered the subtle body, prana body or energy self. We talked about awakening the *nadis* or energy channels in previous chapters.
- *Manamaya Kosha*: this is the mind; it is related to emotions, thoughts and any mental processes.
- *Vijnanamaya Kosha*: the wisdom or intellect sheath; here there is discernment, and it is linked to the sympathetic nervous system. You can refer to it as higher mind.
- *Anandamaya Kosha*: the bliss state or sheath; this comes closest to the experience of joy and contentment and the soul.

This concept makes sense as you start to delve deeper into your true nature or soul. The soul is non-changing and exists in all of us according to Ayurveda. The *Atman* or *Buddhi* aspect exists in every cell according to Ayurveda. So even though we may have our own unique makeup of *pitta*, *kapha* and *vata* cell differentiation according to how we came into this world, there is also a changeless soul aspect that connects all of us. This is a deep and beautiful concept that can set you free when you embrace it. This idea is thousands of years old (that we know of) and may just be timeless.

Wow, all this soul talk in a chapter on sleep and decompressing for the day! This is being taught in spiritual learning centers all around the world and can help you realize that you are not limited to your body. You are not this body; you are way more.

I think you can see that you have a lot of resources in your Ayurvedic tool kit to slip into a deep, restful sleep. This will allow your innate intelligence to repair and restore your body as you sleep. You may find that your dreams become lighter or less. The situations in your dreams may become more pleasant. You can tap into creative energies and even experience dreamless sleep. This is all within the realm of possibility. Now let's explore some energy points in the body that can help you manage your self-care and get more out of a regular massage.

CHAPTER 10

Energy Points and Marma Massage

"Energy cannot be created or destroyed; it can only be changed from one form to another."
– Albert Einstein

All of life is energy in motion, and Ayurveda relies on yogic knowledge to classify the body's energy systems. We have all heard of chakras, or wheels of energy, that exist in the body in seven different locations. Let's explore the chakras for a moment. They are considered energy wheels that radiate from the body in a spinning motion like a wheel. The word chakra means "wheel" or "disc" in Sanskrit. It refers to the physical, mental and spiritual aspects of the energy emanating from that center. Although this may not fit into everyone's belief system, it is worth considering so that you can have a deeper understanding of your yoga practice. Since we can't measure a chakra well because it crosses the various sheaths or koshas in the body, it is best to just know where they are in the body and what they refer to.

The seven chakras are:

1. The Crown Chakra (Sahasrara): It represents higher consciousness and is considered by most yogis to be the place where the divine consciousness and illuminating super-conscious thoughts enter the body. Color: white.
2. Third Eye Chakra (Ajna): This is the seat of psychic energy, intuition and perception. Color: purple.
3. Throat Chakra (Visshudha): This is located in the throat area and is connected to communication and expression of oneself. Often associated with blue, although colors may vary according to the interpretation.
4. Heart Chakra (Anahata): Located in the chest and represents compassion and heart-centeredness. Associated with the color green.
5. Solar Plexus (Manipura): Located in the upper abdominal area. This chakra is associated with a person's confidence and outer expression in the world. Color: yellow.
6. Sacral Chakra (Svadisthana): Located in the lower abdominal area and is connected with sexual and creative energy. Color: orange, although this can vary.
7. Root Chakra (Muladhara): This chakra is at the base of the spine and is related to groundedness and stability. It is a very primal energy center, and the color is red.

Are the chakras real, you may ask? I can say that as an intuitive healer I feel connected to *ajna* chakra, third eye, and a*nahata*, heart center, as I am both an intellectual and a heart-centered person. I don't teach the chakras in my Ayurvedic consultations, but a good working knowledge of them is important for anyone practicing yogic postures. They can serve as focal points during meditation where you can direct your focus on any of these chakras while meditating. I have had many profound experiences focusing on the chakras in meditation. As you become more intuitive and aware in your meditative and yoga practice, you may have the same experience.

Another energy concept I have mentioned is the subtle *nadis* or energy channels in the body. They are activated with pranayama or breathing exercises. There are said to be 72,000 *nadis* or subtle channels in the body, and I outlined three of the main *nadis*: Sushumna, Ida and Pingala. Prana or vital energy flows through the *nadis*. Our goal in Ayurveda is to boost our prana (through breathing exercises and proper diet) and to boost our digestive *agni*. We explored how the three main *nadis* play a big role in pranayama because they work on the sympathetic/parasympathetic nervous systems in the body as well as the central nervous system.

So now let's look at energy pressure points called marma points. Marma means "secret" or "essence" in Sanskrit. Physiologically it refers to the junction of different types of tissues like tendons, ligaments, bones and muscles. In Ayurveda we consider the different sheaths or koshas of the energy body, so marma point acupressure is designed to stimulate and balance the physical, spiritual and energetic dimensions in healing and wellness. It is similar to acupressure points but different, and marma points appear to predate acupuncture. Marma points can be used during self-massage or when massaging others to balance energies and to simply relax. Throughout time medicated oils were used in a therapeutic context to balance these marma points and a person's dosha. For self-massage we can use certain types of oils (based on dosha) as well as essential oils.

Many of the major Ayurvedic texts refer to 107 marma points, yet the total number of primary marmas is 51 because many of the marmas exist on both sides. We will explore how to use the most practical everyday marma points for self-massage as part of a daily or nightly ritual. Many marmas are on the limbs of the body, so a morning marma massage ritual might have you making circular movements with your hands over points in and around your ears, jaw, third eye area (between the eyebrows) and along and around the neck and upper and lower arms. You can get creative with this and, most of all, have fun while you are doing it.

Let's create a marma point massage routine where we will massage the neck, jaw and various points around the head. Then we will massage up and down both the underside and outside of the elbows, forearms, hands and wrists. We'll use circular movements as we do this. You can perform this for 10-15 minutes as a mini-spa gift to yourself as part of a daily ritual. So, let's get familiar with a few key marma points that will be helpful to know for self-massage.

There are 107 marma points. You do not have to know all of them, but look at the illustration below so you can see where they are:

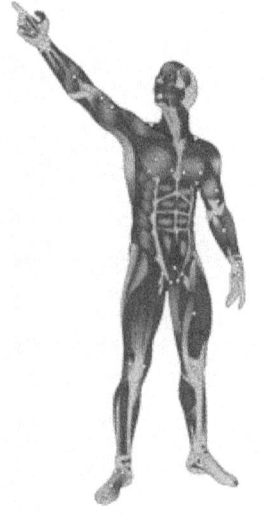 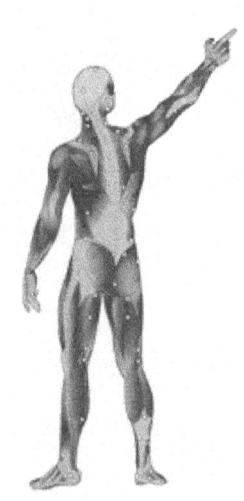

MARMA ENERGY POINTS

Marma points in Head Area (Shira):

- Third Eye Marma (Stapany): Located directly between the eyebrows. This is where the bridge of the nose meets the forehead. Touch this area so that you can feel where the

point is. It can be palpated when you have a sinus headache. It is said that this marma stimulates the pituitary gland.
- *Phana* Marma: This is located below the lower part of the eye socket in line with the center of the eye. Another great point to know to relieve sinus tension.
- *Shringatica* Marma: Located at the bottom of the cheekbone and directly below the pupil. Touch this area to become familiar with it.
- *Manya* Marma: Directly below the earlobe and the jawbone. As you can imagine, this marma is great for releasing jaw tension and has a rejuvenating effect on the body, especially when used with a nice carrier oil and a soothing essential oil.
- *Sankhya* Marma: This is located in the indentation directly behind the earlobe. Massaging this area is said to balance the thyroid gland.
- *Ansa* Marma: This is one-half inch below the base of the skull or about one-half inch out from either side of the spine. Since we tend to hold tension in our neck this is a great point to know.

Marma Points in the Arm and Hand Area:

- *Uru* Marma: Located on the upper arm at the midpoint between the elbow and the shoulder. This pressure point will relieve tension in the tricep/deltoid area, which can sometimes be knotted. This will unblock the energy flow here.
- *Kurpara* Marma: Located in the inner part of elbow joint in the hollow space that you find when you bend your arm. We tend to store tension in our arms and this needs to be released.
- *Gulpha* Marma: Upper part of the forearm just below the elbow.

- *Vataka* Marma: Located on the dorsal side of the hand in the saddle joint that is the thumb. This can provide relief to hand issues related to poor posture and sitting at the computer keyboard incorrectly.
- *Manibandha* Marma: Located at the wrist joint on the back of the hand.
- *Kukundara* Marma: Located on the back of the hand between the thumb and the index finger.

So, let's go over these points in English just to get the mechanics and to start gently massaging them; start by touching them:

Space between eyebrows

Below the lower part of the eye socket

Bottom of the cheekbone

Directly below the earlobe and the jawbone

The indentation behind the earlobe

One-half inch below the skull about a half an inch out from the spine on either side

Then move to arm area:

Upper arm midpoint between the elbow and the shoulder on lateral side of the body

Inner part of elbow joint in the hollow

Upper part of forearm below the elbow again on the lateral side

Back of the hand at the thumb joint

Wrist joint groove on the back of the hand

Back of the hand between the thumb and the index finger

Now let's put together a simple carrier oil and mix in a few drops of essential oil.

Sample Carrier Oils:

Almond Oil: nice, light oil

Jojoba Oil: another light oil made from a southwestern U.S shrub

Coconut Oil: great cooling oil for *pitta* types

Sample Essential Oils:

Lavender: very relaxing and calming

Eucalyptus: excellent for respiratory system

Peppermint: has a cooling effect

Rose: promotes relaxation and very good for the skin

Ginger oil: can be used for muscle and joint pain

Find an oil that you have used on your skin or that you are not allergic to. Choose the same for the essential oil. Know that you have many varieties of carrier oils, including sesame, and an endless variety of essential oils. Please consult with a marma massage expert and an Ayurvedic expert for guidance on particular conditions you may have going on. But for a daily example of a 15-minute quick marma massage ritual, I choose jojoba oil, lavender and rose. I mix a few drops of lavender and rose essential oils into the jojoba and mix it well. Then I begin in gentle circular strokes to massage the points above, taking note where I might need to spend a little extra time. But generally, you travel in circular movements with both hands on the head, face and neck and then of course alternating hands for the arms. As you become more familiar with the points, you can add the back, the tummy and the legs. It is highly recommended to have a certified marma massage therapist give you a nice full-body massage working on all the marma points. He or she will also mix the massage oil and essential oil according to your dosha and what you have going on that day.

Marma point self-massage can be a nice ritual to add to your wake-up routine, even if you have to get up an hour earlier in order to do it. You can do it by yourself or with your partner. Let's explore what a daily ritual would look like. Ritual in Sanskrit is called *dinacharya*, and it is a pretty cool way to start the day. "Din" means day and "charya" means to follow. The daily routine would consist of good hygiene, a healthy diet, moderate exercise and a healthy outlook on life. In the course of every day, according to Ayurveda there are two cycles of change: one occurs from 6 a.m. to 6 p.m. and the other occurs from 6 p.m. to 6 a.m. Within each cycle there are 4-hour time periods that are dominated by either *pitta*, *kapha* or *vata*. Chances are you will be doing your daily routine during *kapha* time or somewhere from 6 a.m. to 10 a.m.

A day can start with marma point massage for 15-20 minutes. If you have a sinus issue, use some eucalyptus in the massage oil and massage the sinus points carefully on the face. If you have a diffuser, turn it on and breathe in the beneficial essential oil. Then take a shower or bath with all natural products to rinse the oil off. Have some hot tea with herbs or hot water with lemon. Practice some pranayama or breathing exercises for 15 minutes. Then do some light yoga stretches that work for your body and dosha type. Do at least 25 minutes if you can, just to get into the routine of a morning ritual. Have a healthy breakfast and start your day with gratitude for all there is. If you do just a little every day, it will become a habit. You will always come back to it. You can do a combo daily ritual of a little meditation, yoga nidra, hatha yoga and self-massage. Put together a simple routine that you can blend into your daily life. If you miss a day, just know that you can always come back to it.

When you want a full-body massage with marma point activation, then order an *abhyanga* massage from the Ayurvedic massage therapist. This is a full-body massage with long strokes performed with oil and herb formulation according to dosha. They may sprinkle a little essential oil in too. It is one of my personal favorites and is excellent for dosha balancing.

We are very fortunate to have options when it comes to our health. Marma points are used in all kinds of Ayurvedic massage. Another massage that is great for the doshas is a head massage called *Shirodhara*. It should be given by a trained Ayurvedic practitioner and will be done with oils and herbs or essential oils that will benefit dosha issues you may have going on. I would like to mention again the two different contexts under which the term dosha will be used. When you understand this, you will know more than the average person about how Ayurvedic knowledge and medicine works. The first context is dosha as constitution, or *prakriti*; the second is dosha as an imbalance, or *vikriti*. Let's explore the differences for a moment.

Dosha as constitution or *prakriti* refers to the inherent nature of the body that is decided at conception. It is your dosha that we determine in your first consultation and it will be used to inform you and to help you in deciding how to nourish it properly. It does not change for the whole life of the individual and is one of the seven types that were mentioned in Chapter 4:

- *Vata*
- *Pitta*
- *Kapha*
- *Vata-Pitta*
- *Pitta-Kapha*
- *Vata-Kapha*
- *Vata-Kapha-Pitta*

There is another meaning of dosha as imbalance in the body and this will be used to describe what you have going on that is problematic. Dosha as imbalance or *vikriti* is a situation where there is a problem related to your dosha. The imbalances can occur mostly because of lifestyle, stress, diet, your environment or a particular health condition. Ayurvedic physicians can go many layers deep in treating more serious imbalances. Here the dosha terms will be used to describe problems within the body. An Ayurvedic expert will give you a health diagnosis to determine what imbalances are presenting in the body. If it is beyond their scope of practice, they will refer you to and work in conjunction with an Ayurvedic physician. Typically, in the United States, an Ayurvedic physician would either be an allopathic doctor with an integrative practice in Ayurvedic medicine or a naturopath with an integrated practice in Ayurvedic medicine. The formal training institutions for Ayurvedic medicine are in India, and it is not yet recognized as medicine in the United States, although the clinical research is there to back up the science.

As a lifelong yoga teacher, yogic science advocate and certified Ayurvedic consultant, I have been helping my clients to lead healthier, happier lives while nourishing their families. This has allowed many of them to attain peak performance levels in their lives or to boost their health in order to heal their own bodies.

Let's explore the head massage called *Shirodhara* next. *Shirodhara* is an Ayurvedic therapy that consists of the pouring of a therapeutic liquid (usually hot oil and herbs according to dosha imbalances) on the forehead of a person who is lying down in a supine position on a massage table. In Sanskrit, *shir* is head and *dhara* means flow. This is a very relaxing treatment and has a tremendous grounding benefit for the person receiving it. Your eyes will be covered while you are receiving it and it typically lasts for 30 minutes to an hour. The third eye center, or *ajna* chakra is an area of focus and clients report feeling refreshed and balanced afterward with a high level of energy. Clients have reported sleeping better after this treatment and the oils used can nourish and balance the pH of the skin. The overall health benefits are tremendous. Although this technique may not be suitable for everyone, I can say that when I received it, I kept the oil in my hair the rest of the day and felt fantastic.

Ayurvedic massage can be a deeply detoxing experience. The detoxing formulas used during the massage experience are custom tailored to the client. It can take many forms. *Svedhana* in Ayurvedic medicine is another spa favorite and involves the inducement of sweating in a controlled environment with steam and herbs. It usually takes place in a pre-sterilized sweat tent, where your head can stick out on one end or you can put your whole body in. It can also be performed with hot compresses with herbs that are applied to the body to induce sweating. It is recommended to consult with an Ayurvedic expert before undergoing any of the therapies so that you have a working sense of which treatment works best for you.

These treatments can be seen as luxurious in many ways because of the deep effects on the body. Ayurvedic knowledge applied to spa-like treatments will easily become the wave of the future. Ayurveda, because of its esoteric nature, has been tricky to understand, but when you see that it is a whole system of health care, including amazing skincare, you will probably fall in love with the benefits. The dietary benefits will take a little focus and discipline, but the benefits will far outweigh the effort. So, enjoy this exploration into the world of botanical and medicinal bliss that is truly the art and science of Ayurveda. Health is the true wealth here and you deserve it!

CHAPTER 11

Let Excellent Health Be Your Guide

You will never be defined by any health condition, and you can easily take your health into your own hands with Ayurveda. Most people don't realize that their health is always changing and transforming. They are never stuck in time unless things are terminal, and even then I have seen people rally in incredible ways. When I think of the number of relatives and clients who have put the future of their health in the hands of someone or something outside of themselves, it is staggering. I had a relative who started to develop a liver tumor at age 50, after taking a popular prescription drug for lowering cholesterol. I watched as she slowly deteriorated over the course of five years. She lost her hair and then became weak from chemotherapy. She didn't connect the dots that this drug may have been causing her health problems, but it was the only thing she was doing differently. She never stopped taking it and whatever her doctor told her, she obeyed without challenging it. She passed away within five years. I couldn't believe it and I was very young at the time. I knew that there was more she could have done on her end.

I've seen too many people ignore the elephant in the room, which is usually a health problem that they don't want to talk about. Many times, these people think it's best to keep the problem to themselves so that they won't burden anyone. I have a friend who recently passed away at the age of 44 from colon cancer. She did not want to tell anyone until the last weeks of her life when everything was falling apart. At that point she finally let her parents know and it was way too late. Maybe she could have chosen a complementary Ayurvedic therapy to the traditional chemotherapy and that might have boosted her immune system. Maybe she could have expressed herself earlier on, but in the end, nothing was done.

When you start taking your health into your own hands using Ayurvedic knowledge, you will have a treasure trove of health possibilities. You can start to balance your own nervous system and get rid of anxiety with pranayama breathing exercises, yoga exercises and yoga nidra. You can cook up meals, smoothies and teas that energize your system instead of depleting you. Where else will you be able to engage all your senses in the process? We are here on earth for a reason, and why not live it up by using all five senses (seeing, feeling, tasting, smelling and hearing) when you are preparing meals? This will create a natural healing environment in your own kitchen no matter how busy you are.

When you start to add a healthy daytime and nighttime ritual to your busy life along with the amazing tips on health care, you will become unstoppable. I found over the years that even the busiest of clients were able to fit in a little Ayurvedic boost each day. Whether it's meditating, self-massage, cooking, pranayama exercises or yoga nidra, where there is a will there is a way.

You can easily perform pranayama exercises on the go. My client Faith insisted that she had no time for breathing exercises, so I had her do simple breath-retention exercises in the car on the way to work. Once she stopped getting in her own way with the "no time" excuse, she started pulling over on the side of the road and doing a few rounds of alternate nostril breathings (*nadi shodhana*). She said it really helped her let go of anxiety around her commute and brightened her day. Another client uses some of the breathing techniques on the train and said she just focuses on her chakras and goes within. She actually said that she used her commute to become better at meditation and yoga nidra. You can too! There is plenty of time in a day if you know where to look.

As you put together all seven of the Ayurvedic recommendations I have given you, you will start to feel more energy from the foods you eat and create a new eating pattern that will serve you and your loved ones for a long time. You will be delivering more oxygen to your cells through pranayama exercises and also through the nutritious herbs, spices and foods that you will be adding to your meals. You will be mindful of exercises that work for you and your dosha and that stimulate the energy systems of your body. You will also have a tremendous resource with yoga poses that work for your body type. This in turn will allow you to increase your range of motion and prevent injury. You will have an edge in any other exercise classes that you take by knowing yoga exercises. As your body becomes more alkaline and less acidic by resting your neurology and preparing healthy meals, you will have the most valuable health insurance, all from the comfort of your own home. The detoxing of your cells and your life will occur naturally because of following these Ayurvedic ideas. You can experiment with essential oils to boost your immune system and to enhance your massages. Your life will become more sensual by nature with health as its cornerstone.

Your awareness will be more fine-tuned by knowing about the body's elaborate energy systems that no one ever told you about. The *nadis*, the marma points and the boosting of prana and digestive *agni* are all a part of your vocabulary now. You will become your own doctor in many ways as you learn how to make yourself feel better naturally. Your awareness of the five koshas or sheaths of existence will allow you to realize that you are way more than a physical body. This concept takes some yoga practitioners many years to realize.

When you start to see each day as an opportunity to create a ritual for your health, you will look forward to getting up earlier each day, or setting aside "sacred space" time each day. This is setting an intention for health excellence, and you will be glad you did. This is an expression of self-love that will allow you to give more in the world if that is your goal. Your nightly ritual can become an adventure in self-awareness, rejuvenation, calmness and creativity. The yoga nidra can be used to set positive intentions in your transformational life as you observe your body from a unique perceptual position.

When my client Leanna started to apply some of the pranayama exercises, yoga nidra and self-massage ideas to her daily life, it started to transform her relationship with her husband. Her whole sense of health and wellness changed for the better. Leanna is a busy CEO of a small private equity firm and her ideas about the world were mostly negatively charged. This was hidden behind a belief that she would never be good enough and that her employees resented her because she was a woman. We worked through this therapeutically through Vedic counseling about her role in the world, her obligation to her family and her view of herself. In conjunction with ego-strengthening, the Ayurvedic applications became the icing on the cake for Leanna. She started to be more compassionate to her employees and developed a strong appreciation for herself. This allowed her to indulge in yoga nidra exploration, massages and pranayama. She said she started to feel like a different person and this in turn spilled over to her marriage, which was going through a rough patch. She was able to share some of the massage and cooking ideas with her husband and this brought them closer together.

When Renata came to me, she had tried to lose weight on her own and nothing worked. She was at a stage in her life where losing weight was difficult. She needed to lose twenty pounds to fit into some of her old clothes and ideally forty pounds to feel otherworldly. One of the first things I did as her Ayurvedic consultant was to manage expectations so that she could tune into gradual weight loss that she could control. We found some *kapha* imbalances which are very common in people trying to lose weight. She really got to know her dosha well through the consultation and started to realize that the tendency to gain weight was being driven by her natural constitution (heaviness, easygoing stride in life, nothing too urgent) and also by other potential factors such as hormonal imbalances, environmental influences, a clearly sluggish digestive system, and fatty liver. I worked in conjunction with an Ayurvedic physician with her and she has now lost a total of 25 pounds over the course of 10 weeks, and is still counting. We were able to put together a natural herbal protocol and eliminate some of the digestive stressors in Renata's life.

I have been working with my client Michael for a few years now. His improvements have occurred over time at his own pace as he brought many elements in his life forward to make the space to follow an Ayurvedic protocol. He was very ADD and was taking drugs for this. This information did not come out in the beginning of our working together. As I tuned into his *vata* (airy nature), I had to ask is this truly biochemical or is this a learned behavior? It was revealed over time that this appeared to be a learned behavior. His doctor approved of the work we were doing, which always helps the client. As he was able to gradually wean himself off the medication, he would occasionally slip back, but we took it slow. We worked through some of the family problems it was creating for him. We got to a point where he was letting himself be loved, especially by himself. As this happened and I asked, "How good are you willing to allow yourself to feel?," something inside of him started to click. He started to take serious interest in his *vata* imbalances and worked to correct them through dietary and lifestyle changes. As I layered in yogic exercises, yoga nidra, pranayama and regular Ayurvedic massages, he became so much more grounded and confident. When Michael decided that enough was enough with abusing his health and that he was no longer in denial, miracles began to happen. Here they happened in the eleventh hour when he was feeling at his most vulnerable.

I found as I shared Ayurveda with my family and friends that the world can benefit from this knowledge. It doesn't have to be lofty or complicated if it is explained in a way that makes it accessible for everyone. That is my goal in sharing this knowledge. There is so much opportunity to boost your health and prevent health problems before they become more difficult. I was always proactive with my own personal Ayurvedic consultations so that I knew what to look for and what to focus on in my own health. This allowed me to get ahead of some issues that might have become problematic down the line. My issues were a *kapha* imbalance (sinus) and difficulty in metabolizing sugar properly. Fortunately, this was revealed by a biochemistry profile of my metabolism, which is a great proactive test for anyone to take. It measured certain physiological aspects of my metabolism like Krebs cycle, micronutrients and cellular methylation.

Wherever you are on your health journey, you can have similar successes that all my clients have had when you have the desire to live your healthiest life. The resources that Ayurveda provides are not complicated and they do not cost very much. If you are used to buying lots of supplements, sports drinks or green drinks, you can save yourself a lot of money. If you are eating the worst foods and not taking care of yourself, you will also save money. Gee, maybe that is why these ideas are not as widely promoted as they should be. Just know that it's never too late to start as long as you have the will and the means.

If you need to lose weight like my client Renata, and you are open to adding some simple changes to your daily routine and meal preparation, you can have the same results. Because we are treating your health from the inside out, you will be way ahead of most people. If you need to let go of a medication or a situation that is holding your health back and you learn tools that empower your health, you will be successful. If you feel overwhelmed with responsibility but want to take ownership of your health and life, you can have similar results to Leanna. An added perk for her was that her marriage improved naturally.

By following the strategies I have described for Ayurvedic health, you will be able to experience excellent health with the high possibility that you will increase your life span. But you will need to take action, so I recommend that you book an Ayurvedic consultation appointment as soon as possible and learn about your dosha. Then tune into the areas where your health is showing signs of blockage or sluggishness and follow the recommendations from the consultation, which will include herbal and dietary recommendations. The idea in Ayurveda is that all or most diseases originate in the mouth and digestive system. So, you will be given sound nutritional advice on how to get rid of *ama* and inflammation in the body and how to restore and energize areas that might be lacking in your health. You will have the tools (that should be taught in every school) that show how to care for your digestive health and absorption of nutrients.

Next, sign up for a yoga class that complements your dosha. Since there are many styles of yoga, I recommend finding one that matches more closely the kind of dosha boost you may need. For example, if you are a *kapha* person and may need to lose weight, you might want to consider the faster-moving classes. You may need to avoid classes with excess heat. If you are a driven *pitta* personality, you may need something more conducive to elongating your muscles and slowing you down while still being interesting. Sivananda or Iyengar styles might be recommended. If you have any questions, feel free to reach out to me at the email address in this book or in our Facebook group.

You should create areas in your home that support both your daytime and your nighttime rituals. Start to clear the space in your kitchen and make room for your new foods in their glass jars. Get an electric pressure cooker if you really want to explore the world of legumes and legume dishes. Make sure you have plenty of glass jars to house legumes, rice, spices and herbs. Start to really know your kitchen as well as the new herbs, spices and cooking recipes. You will become a great food warrior and your ideas about eating and digestion will naturally evolve and change for the better. It's quality and not quantity that matters in Ayurveda.

Book a massage with an Ayurvedic massage expert and choose one that is based on your dosha. If you need more grounding, then get a *Shirodhara* or head massage. If you need a good detox, then ask for a *svedhana* or sweat massage. Go to an Ayurvedic center with a great reputation. Most of the places I have been to are fine, but please double-check their credentials. If you need to move things around a bit in your body, then get a full-body massage or abhyanga. There will always be endless surprises with what a good

Ayurvedic consultant can offer you in terms of ointments, herbs and skin care products that you can take home with you.

Ayurveda teaches that when it comes to skin and hair care products, you should never use anything on your body that you can't safely ingest. This will bring awareness to the amount of chemicals that you may have lying around your bathroom. Do a bathroom check and see if you can find natural skin and body care products. This can be difficult when it comes to hair these days, but Ayurvedic experts are big on natural henna, brahmi oil and other natural products for hair care. The weird thing is, in these modern times you still won't be able to dye your hair naturally, except with henna. Oh well... Did you know that a great natural facial scrub can be made with just oatmeal and plain natural yogurt? There are many Ayurvedic hacks that are naturally healthy for both skin and hair care.

Explore yoga nidra and your nighttime ritual to the point where you make it a work of art. Create an environment where sacred rest can take place in a peaceful environment. Otherwise, you may be giving away those precious hours to the gods of worry, agitation and overstimulation. There will always be tomorrow to conquer the world, but you might find that you are conquering your inner world by doing yoga nidra exercises, setting up your room and having all electronic devices off. I have every bit of faith that you can be as successful as my clients have been in achieving excellent health. Excellent health is relative to how we have been with our health, and there is always room to improve it. Ayurveda shows the way.

CHAPTER 12

Create Community with Your Ayurveda Knowledge

When you first started reading *Ayurveda: Health Is Wealth*, I bet you started asking yourself, "Just what is Ayurveda?" As you started reading and absorbing the health ideas, I am sure you realized that you can do it and that it's not as hard as you thought. I can assure you that as we go through the challenging times ahead, you will need all the health support you can get. You will also need a sense of peace and calm for your health going into future times. Stressors will be coming at you from all angles, so you best be prepared. The media will be trying to scare the bejesus out of you so that you start stocking up on unnecessary prescription drugs and the next new shiny object in holistic over-supplementation.

The pharmaceutical companies create some of the most seductively crafted ads in the industry with catchy jingles and great actors. Don't fall for it. It is the most insidious form of hypnosis there is, as the tonal inflection drops when the commercial announcer is describing all the bad things your "perfect drug" can do to your system: may cause suicidal thoughts, sudden stroke or death, etc. Why would we gamble with these risk factors? I don't know about you, but I will put my money on natural healing methods from an ancient source anytime over some big pharmaceutical company. They even have drug they try to sell you that help your current anti-depressant work so that you do not feel as depressed. Come on, we are not that stupid.

I say it's okay to enjoy the catchy jingles, but don't buy what they are selling. The United States is one of the few countries in the world where drug companies can pitch directly to the consumer. As of this writing, New Zealand is the other country that allows this. This is no joke because people are being hypnotized into an over reliance on drugs and conditions without knowing what hit them.

The GMO companies in agribusiness are making sure that they are maximizing profits and minimizing choices in the food industry. If large multi-national GMO companies cannot even make a safe weed killer, you can bet they didn't follow best practices in introducing genetically modified seeds into the food supply. We are getting hit at a rapid speed by chemically altered foods. We are seeing a struggling environment where air and ground pollution is running rampant and where our fish in the oceans are ingesting plastics. There is a lot to be concerned about, especially when cardiovascular disease and diabetes statistics are so incredibly high in the United States.

According to the American Heart Association's statistics from 2019, about half the population of adults in the U.S has some form of heart disease. It was reported in 2021 that 88 million adults had pre-diabetes in the U.S., and this often leads to type 2 diabetes if not managed properly. Also, about 10.5 percent of the population in 2021, or 34.2 million people, had full-blown diabetes. These numbers are staggering and only on the rise. Something is clearly not working in our system of health.

I presented seven steps in Ayurveda that will clearly help you actualize better health. If you introduce them gradually into your existing lifestyle, your health will prosper. The seven steps are:

1. Know your dosha or constitution by getting an Ayurvedic consultation. Apply the knowledge to create a custom system of health care for yourself that is balancing, nourishing and cleansing.
2. Exercise for your dosha. The spine needs to be strengthened and lengthened. The movements need to occur in different directions or planes of movement. Have your Ayurvedic consultant design a posture-specific routine that makes you feel wonderful.
3. Learn pranayama breathing exercises and sprinkle them throughout your day. The increased oxygen will have a cleansing and balancing effect and you will experience more clarity. Take the time to learn the biomechanics of the breathing exercises and then just show up and do them.
4. Transform your kitchen into a healing health laboratory. Clear the space and let go of old overly processed foods that no longer serve you. Start adding legumes and grains to your diet and become familiar with various herbs and spices that nourish you.
5. Know which foods promote digestion and use them to your advantage. Make homemade yogurt or get a yogurt maker, and do a one a day a week fast with a detox smoothie. Prepare some of the easy-to-follow recipes and add them to your family's diet.
6. Learn about yoga nidra and create a sleep ritual and sanctuary for yourself. Make nighttime another universe in which to explore restorative sleep. Make sure to take hot baths, use essential oils and have all electronics off. Have fun with this!

7. Do regular self-massage with basic marma point knowledge and get an Ayurvedic massage. Get an *abhyanga* (full-body), *Shirodhara* (head massage) and/or *svedhana* (sweat massage), which all have nourishing herbs and oils for the skin, hair and soul.

The first time I ever received a *Shirodhara* massage was at a yoga center in the Caribbean and it was the most gorgeous feeling! First, you are at sea level with fresh oxygen-rich air. There is plenty of time to rest after the massage too. It was wonderful to allow my scalp to absorb the dosha-specific herbs and oils because I did not have to work afterward. I could let these nutrients get absorbed into my skin and I felt fantastic! It worked on all systems and koshas in my body, and it made the yoga classes I was taking that much easier.

But you do not have to be on a beach in the Caribbean. Your next massage is just a phone call away and might involve a drive, but it's worth it. As long as you know that your massage therapist is well qualified in Ayurveda, you can start to enjoy the benefits right away.

No matter what health concerns you have, Ayurvedic knowledge and consultants will help you to heal them. Remember my client Melody in Chapter 1, who was experiencing swollen feet and ankles? The remedy for this needed to be a multi-pronged approach that included prescriptive yoga poses, pranayama exercises, adding good, nutritious Ayurvedic meals to her diet and improving her sleep habits. She started to have a whole new sense of who she was. She did matter and she did have the power to change her habits. You can have the same amazing results that Melody did.

Maybe you have fatty liver issues like my client Kathy did, or a job that is wreaking havoc on your weight and your sense of balance like Michael. All these situations can be changed for the better through the application of the seven principles I've outlined in Ayurveda. You will feel more hope and be able to create health goals for excellence and peak performance if that is your desired outcome. Once you start tuning into the inner subtle workings of your own magnificent body, you will realize that at any given moment there is an Ayurvedic health boost that you can give yourself. You will become unstoppable like so many of my clients.

The seven steps I have outlined here will give you a panoramic view of your health that you will not find anywhere else. You won't find it outside of yourself. All your answers are within, and Ayurveda helps you unlock the door. There will always be an action you can take to improve your health, and this will help you to be more in the moment too. The mindset is built into the system. Even if you were to take two of the ideas and start implementing them today, say knowing your dosha and performing pranayama, you will notice a difference.

I want you to view this as a fun challenge to implement all seven of the ideas here and to have some fun while doing them. I have to say, in the beginning, not everyone is comfortable with pranayama exercises. But you will get used to it and know your body better. You will see how different your body can be every day and tune into areas where you hold tension. The key here is to "do a little every day." Don't make it a project, just make it irresistibly easy to insert into your daily routine. When you start doing a little every day, stick to it and you will enjoy the benefits.

Just the idea of taking quality time out of your day for you is an act of incredible self-love. You will have more energy to give back to others and those you love. You can think of these steps as an Ayurvedic shopping list. Let's see…the first thing you want to do is book an Ayurvedic consultation with an expert and get sound feedback on your dosha. Then you can put that into action right away. Maybe you will be buying a new herb for tea, or some other wonderful herbs that are specifically designed for what you have going on right now. Great!

Then you will have knowledge about the types of exercises that will be best for your constitution, and you can start practicing some of the exercises at home, in the studio or both. When shopping for a yoga class, find one that complements your energy. A tense person who is maybe *pitta* dosha will not benefit from a strenuous fast-moving class, because they need to slow down. An overweight person with a *kapha* imbalance will need to be up and moving more and will benefit from spinal movements that stimulate the endocrine system. There will always be so much to explore here. I also teach anti-gravity classes, so inverted yoga postures can work beautifully on some metabolic issues. Everything is performed gently at first and the intensity can be increased gradually.

Then you will start to make the hand positions like chin mudra and Vishnu mudra part of a regular pranayama or breathing practice. Yogic breathing exercises or pranayama are a secret weapon of yogis, and many performers use them in order to increase their endurance or performance charisma. Once upon a time I attended a play that was written by yogic master Sri Chinmoy and the performers were all yogis or yoga students. Their stage presence was phenomenal and very charismatic. The play was compelling, the performers had incredible posture and their voices were very resonant.

Clinical research has shown that pranayama exercises are beneficial for treating neurological disorders, but there is still more to explore about breath retention, exhalation and bellows exercises. These exercises are an integral part of any pranayama routine and can contribute to longevity and outstanding health. We know in the animal kingdom that slower breathing patterns (meaning longer inspiration and exhalation times) do seem to contribute to an animal's lifespan, in the case of elephants and turtles, for example. This is directly related to metabolism and might be an indication that taking things in their stride will contribute to a long life. When you practice pranayama techniques you will see measurable results in your holding times, and this is very motivating. You will be using pranayama to boost your health, but the benefits of practicing different pranayama techniques extend far beyond even health.

As you clean the space in your kitchen for new foods and cooking utensils, you can breathe easy knowing that these foods will always be easier to digest and absorb than regular foods. You can enjoy cooking with an endless variety of herbs and spices that will make it a very interesting journey. You can get creative sharing these meals with the people you love. Since taste is such an integral part of the cooking process, you can mix and match to make them tasty and appealing. You can also enjoy engaging the five senses, which is another integral part of any Ayurvedic kitchen. The smells, sounds of herbs crackling and the sights of different foods are all a part of this Ayurvedic cooking choreography.

You can look forward to creatively winding down at the end of a long day into sleep or yoga nidra as part of a restorative ritual. This will enhance your creative juices and give you more peace of mind about your sleep habits. There are so many untapped resources within you and your environment when you retreat for the night. Darkness for sleep can be great for the adrenal glands that are largely on fight-or-flight during an overly hectic day. You will start mastering your ability to relax and to sleep in style. You can take a yoga nidra class and apply the wisdom of the teachings to your meditation practice.

And of course, you can indulge in a high-quality Ayurvedic massage for the head or the whole body where your body can soak in the soothing herbs and oils. You can top off the massage with a *svedhana* or a sweat tent massage if the Ayurvedic center has one. Or you can create your own steam sauna at home, maybe adding your own essential oils of eucalyptus, peppermint or lavender and rose. Just as there are thousands of herbs and plants to explore in Ayurveda, there are also hundreds of essential oils. You will enjoy learning about all of them.

So now that you know that you can create your own healthy lifestyle with Ayurvedic wisdom, you may want to share it with your community. Many Ayurvedic centers have a supportive community and if you do not find one, then I suggest starting one. One of my clients started one with the kids and teachers in her son's school. Then it gradually developed into a regular program. Kids were being taught about healthy snacks and nutritious meals were served. They became the next generation of Ayurvedic kids.

You can introduce Ayurveda into your work environment too. In an office where caffeine and sugary snacks were the norm, one client started preparing teas and Ayurvedic snacks for the employees. They started asking for more and eventually she turned it into a local business. Ayurveda will always be an educational art, so my client offered classes to teach local businesses about adding Ayurveda to their lunch and snack rooms. Ayurvedic foods are quite inexpensive and very eco-friendly, so the good karma will have a snowball effect when you go forth and teach Ayurveda locally. This contributes to joy and peace of mind.

You can add some of the meals to holiday dinners with family. I make a delicious, festive fruit stew that my family gobbles up during holidays. I also make a healthy raw seed stuffing for my family's turkey, and they love it because it tastes great. The key is in the spices and special herbs. I also make a special vegan loaf with a unique blend of herbs, spices and plants that is a super hit. It tastes like turkey only better, and it took some experimenting to get the recipe just right. Please reach out to me on my website to get that recipe.

The most important thing is that you have options in life for your health and wellness. You do not have to be the victim of a poor healthcare system and food supply. There will always be a way if you are committed. I am committed to my clients and my community to help restore balance to their health and wellness through the knowledge of Ayurveda.

It is the gift that keeps giving and will continue to last for many generations to come. Our nervous systems have taken a toll with modern industrialization and bombardment of conflicting opinions and thoughts on health. It's time to return to basics and beautiful simplicity. Move away from over reliance on a broken healthcare system that is only relevant when something is wrong. Become proactive with your health and you will tap into lasting true wealth. There is nothing more empowering than this!

I am dedicated to helping you in your Ayurvedic journey and have access to a wide variety of resources. I am available for public speaking on the Joys of Ayurveda that is great for corporate wellness and private speaking events. You can book an Ayurvedic consultation with me by reaching out to susan@susan.coach or healthcoach212@gmail.com. Take my Ayurvedic dosha quiz on my website at healthiswealthayurveda.com. I look forward to sharing and educating until Ayurveda is an everyday household word. Till then, stay healthy!

REFERENCES

https://www.mayo.edu/research/faculty/pasricha-pankaj-j-m-b-b-s-m-d/bio-20551507

https://www.ncbi.nlm.nih.gov/pmc/articles/PMC3681046/

https://mnj.journals.ekb.eg/article_295602_043f01b8237553ed5bcdbb86df296ed8.pdf

https://molecularneurodegeneration.biomedcentral.com/articles/10.1186/s13024-023-00632-5

https://www.cdc.gov/obesity/data/prevalence-maps.html

Sandhya T, et al. "Potential of traditional Ayurvedic formulation, Triphala, as a novel anticancer drug." Cancer letters 2006; 231 (2): 206-14

Dr. D. Frawley, Dr. S. Ranade and Dr. A. Lele; *[2003] Ayurveda and Marma Therapy: Energy Points in Yogic Healing;* Twin Lakes, Wisconsin; Lotus Press

L. Lidell, Narayani and G. Rabinovitch; [1983]; *The Sivananda Companion to Yoga;* New York; Simon & Shuster, Inc.

Dr. R. K Sharma and V. B. Dash; Agnivesa's Caraka Samhita: Text with English Translation; Varanasi, India; Chowkhamba Sanskrit Series Office

GLOSSARY OF AYURVEDIC TERMS

Abhyanga: A full-body massage in Ayurveda style (with oils and herbs or essential oils). This also refers to the routine of self-massage.

Adaptogens: Nontoxic herbs, roots and plant extracts that help the body relax and de-stress. They are said to be very therapeutic for the nervous system.

Ajna: The sixth primary chakra or subtle energy center, located between the eyebrows. It is associated with intuition and wisdom.

Ama: A toxic byproduct that can accumulate on the tongue and in the body which is an indicator of poor digestion. In Ayurveda, a buildup of ama can lead to disease.

Amalaki: An Indian fruit also called gooseberry; it balances all three doshas and is immune boosting, anti-inflammatory and excellent for the liver.

Amaranth: There are 60 different species of the amaranth plant that is used as a highly nutritious "pseudo-cereal." It's a plant and not a grain and is used often in vegetarian cookery.

Amla (*Emilia Officinalis*): Another name for Indian gooseberry or amalaki; it is also an adjective to describe the taste called "sour."

Anahata: The fourth primary chakra, located in the chest area and considered an emotional center.

Anandamaya (Kosha): One of the five sheaths of existence that house the soul of an individual according to Vedantic philosophy. This one is innermost and is considered the sheath of bliss. It represents one's highest potential and experiencing this layer can lead to enlightenment.

Annamaya (Kosha): One of the five sheaths or koshas according to the Vedas or Vedantic philosophy. It is the "food sheath" and represents the gross physical body which is the most superficial layer and also the one farthest away from the soul. The various koshas or sheaths vary from the energetic level to the more subtle levels of intellect, mind and pure bliss.

Aromatherapy: The use of essential oils that are aromatic and derived from plants in order to enhance the health of the body, mind and spirit.

Ashtanga Hridaya (Ayurvedic Treatise): One of the most influential ancient treatises on Ayurveda. Written in 500-600CE by Vaghbatam, the text consists of 120 chapters in verse form. The name refers to the eight (*ashta*) limbs (*anga*) of medicine (*hridaya*) and identifies over 700 medicinal plants. It explains their usage and how to formulate them.

Ashwagandha: An ancient medicinal herb that has been used in Ayurveda for over 3,000 years. The roots are rich in alkaloids that have analgesic, anti-inflammatory and antioxidant effects.

Astringent: One of the six tastes (sweet, salty, sour, bitter, astringent and pungent) in Ayurveda. Here astringent can create a tightening, puckering sensation in the mouth usually due to the presence of tannins in the food.

Atman: In Sanskrit, refers to the true self or soul. In Hindu philosophy it is the immortal essence of each living individual and is also referred to as supreme spirit and inverse brahman.

Ayurveda: The holistic system of health care that originated in India over 3,000 years ago. It uses a whole-body approach to integrate mind, body and spirit while enhancing good digestion of foods.

Ayurvedic expert: A person who has an in-depth understanding of Ayurvedic principles like doshas (bioenergies) and *agni* (digestive capacity) that determine one's health in Ayurveda. An Ayurvedic expert will perform diagnostic methods like pulse and tongue analysis along with in-depth questioning about diet, health and presenting health issues. They have received formal training and abide by a code of ethics for the profession.

Bhastrika (Breath Exercise): A pranayama or yogic breathing technique that is sometimes referred to as "bellows breathing." It's a series of quick exhalations as the abdominal muscles contract in and out. It increases oxygen and blood circulation in the body.

Bhibitaki (Terminalia Bellirica): One of the three ingredients in the Ayurvedic formulation Triphala. It consists of the fruits and tree of the plant Terminalia bellirica. It has anti-inflammatory, antiviral, antibacterial and analgesic properties.

Brhattrayi: The three foundational texts in the Vedic tradition that consist of the Rigveda, Yajurveda and Samaveda.

Buddhi: The higher mental functioning of a person in Ayurveda. It is also used to describe the self or pure consciousness.

Carrageenan: A food additive made from red seaweed. It is used as a thickening and texturizing agent in many food products. Its effects on the human digestive system are still being studied.

Carrier Oil: An oil used to dilute essential oils so that it is safe to use on the skin. It is made from the fatty portions of plants. Some examples of carrier oils are jojoba, olive, coconut, avocado, almond, grapeseed, argan and avocado oil.

Cellular Nutrition: Refers to consuming foods that support health and function at the cellular level. This is a focal point for Ayurvedic recipes.

Chakra: Chakra means "wheel" in Sanskrit and refers to the subtle energy centers in the body that are thought of as spinning wheels of energy that allow the flow of prana or energy throughout the body. There are seven major chakras that run from the crown of the head to the base of the spine.

Charak Samhita: An important foundational text in Ayurveda written around 400-200 BCE by the Indian physician Charaka.

Chia Seed (Salvia hispanica): Tiny nutritionally dense seeds that are rich in antioxidants, omega-3 fatty acids, fiber, calcium and trace minerals.

Chin Mudra: A hand position used in meditation, yoga and pranayama exercises. Chin means consciousness and it consists of touching the thumb and forefinger together of both hands.

Chutney: A flavorful condiment that originated in India. It is used to enhance taste and accompany meals. There are many different types, including coconut chutney, tomato chutney, tamarind chutney and mint chutney.

Dosha: There are three doshas that refer to one's constitution or biophysical energies in Ayurveda: *kapha*, *pitta* and *vata*. From a a diagnostic standpoint dosha also can mean a problem in the body and the *kapha*, *pitta* and *vata* terms are used to describe the nature of a condition in the body.

Essential Oil: The oils extracted from the bark, stems, flowers, roots and other parts of a plant that are used to enhance the health of the body, mind and spirit. The most popular oils are rose, lavender, lemon, eucalyptus and tea tree to name a few. Essential oils are known to reduce anxiety, ease depression and boost health. They can be used topically or inhaled for the most part.

Five Elements (Ayurveda): The five elements according to Ayurveda are earth (*Prithvi*), water (*Jala*), fire (*Agni*), air (*Vayu*) and space (*Akasha*).

Ghee: Clarified butter that is made by removing the milk solids from regular butter. It is rich in fat-soluble vitamins A, D, E and K and also contains short chain fatty acids.

Graminae Family: A family of grasses which includes important agricultural crops such as wheat, corn, barley, oats, sugar and sorghum. The focus is on the part of the plant that is used and its nutritional value.

Haritaki (Terminalia Chebula): A medicinal fruit that comes from Asia and India. The fruit is yellowish-green in color and used to treat digestive disorders, coughs, parasites, skin problems and other issues. It contains tannins, is anti-bacterial, anti-inflammatory and antioxidant.

Himalayan Salt: A type of rock salt that is extracted from the Punjab region in the Himalayas that is rich in trace minerals. It is 98% sodium chloride and 2% trace minerals such as calcium, magnesium and potassium.

Ida: One of the three major subtle energy channels (the other two are Pingala and Sushumna), or *nadi* channels. It is accessed through pranayama exercises. It is a channel that governs the left side of the body, the yin or lunar energy. It is connected to the parasympathetic nervous system.

Kamut: An ancient wheat grain that preceded modern wheat which comes from the Khorasan area of the Middle East. It is more easily digestible than regular wheat but does contain gluten.

Kapha: One of the three doshas or constitutions in Ayurveda. It is made of the elements earth and water.

Kasaya (Astringent): One of the six tastes in Ayurveda characterized by a dry, puckering, tight taste. The six tastes are sweet, salty, sour, pungent, bitter and astringent.

Katu (Pungent): One of the six tastes in Ayurveda characterized by a hot, spicy flavor. It can be used to balance *kapha* dosha and enhance digestive fire. Some examples are garlic, onions, spicy peppers, mustard and black pepper.

Kosha: Refers to one of the five sheaths of existence that make up a human being on the physical, spiritual, mental and energetic levels.

Kumbhaka: A pranayama or breathing exercise in yoga that consists of breath retention. The breath is held for a small duration of time either on an inhalation or an exhalation to help build lung capacity and to oxygenate the body.

Lavata (Salty): One of the six tastes in Ayurveda. It is common in sodium chloride (table salt), some seaweeds, sea salt and of course salty foods.

Madhura (Sweet): One of the six tastes in Ayurveda. It consists of the elements earth and water and the taste is said to be grounding and satisfying for the body and the mind. It can be found naturally in fruits and is good in moderation.

Manipura: The solar plexus energy center or chakra. Located in the naval/upper abdominal area in the subtle energy body.

Manomaya: One of the five sheaths or koshas that surround the human body in Vedantic philosophy. This particular sheath is the mental sheath.

Marma Points: Vital points in the body where muscles, ligaments, tendons and blood vessels meet. There are 107 marma points in the body, where applied pressure through massage can facilitate the flow of blood, oxygen and prana throughout the body.

Meditation: In Ayurveda, a mindfulness practice that can involve emptying the mind, focusing on a particular object or chakra, or that can be part of a yoga nidra practice. Its basic aim is to calm the disturbances of the mind in order to facilitate peace and healing.

Muladhara: One of the seven chakras or subtle energy centers of the body. Located at the base of the spine and considered the root chakra. It has to do with survival and stability of the individual.

Mung Beans: A highly nutritious legume with a green covering and yellow interior. They are used a lot in Ayurvedic cooking as they are easy to digest and are rich in protein, magnesium, iron and potassium.

Nadi: A subtle energy in the body. There are said to be over 72,000 subtle energy channels or *nadis* in the body.

Nadi Shodhana: Alternate nostril breathing in yoga and Ayurveda.

Pingala: One of the three main subtle energy channels or *nadis* in the body that run along the spine.

Pitta: One of the three doshas or bioenergy types according to Ayurveda that is made up of fire and water elements.

Pouttika: A type of honey collected by very large bees.

Prana: The vital life force that runs through all living beings. It flows through the many thousands of energy channels of the body and concentrates at the chakras.

Pranamaya: One of the five sheaths or koshas surrounding the body. This refers to the sheath made of prana or vital force energy.

Pranayama: Breath control techniques in Ayurveda and yoga.

Quinoa: A pseudo-cereal that is prepared and eaten like a grain. It is rich in zinc, iron, folate and magnesium.

Rajas: One of the three qualities or *gunas* that make up the mind and which also describes objects and food. Rajas' quality exudes energy, passion, spiciness and excessive activity.

Rasa: "Taste" in Sanskrit; there are six tastes.

Safed Musli (Chlororphytum kborivilianum): Herb in Ayurvedic medicine with white tuberous roots that is a restorative tonic for sexual health and also for managing diabetes.

Sahasrara: The crown chakra that is at the top of the head; considered a thousand-petalled lotus. It is the seat of enlightenment, consciousness and spiritual connection.

Sanskrit: An ancient Indo-Aryan language that is considered one of the oldest languages in the world. It is used in classical Hindu texts.

Satva: The concept of truthfulness in the practice of yoga; one of the ethical principles in yoga (Yamas).

Savasana: Corpse pose in yoga.

Shatavari (Asparagus racemosus): A popular herb in Ayurvedic medicine for female reproductive health that is characterized by woody stems and needle-like leaves.

Shilajit: A tar-like substance that comes from the Himalayas and other mountain ranges. It is formed over time by the decomposition of plants and microbial matter which causes it to ooze out of the rocks when sunlight hits it. It is rich in fulvic acid and minerals and is considered a rejuvenating adaptogen in Ayurveda.

Shirodhara: Derived from the Sanskrit words *shiro* meaning "head" and *dhara* meaning "flow." It's a traditional form of Ayurvedic therapy that involves the continuous pouring of warm oils on the forehead or "third eye" area. It is used for dosha balancing.

Spelt (Triticum spelta): An ancient grain that belongs to the wheat family which is rich in protein, B vitamins, magnesium and iron. It does contain gluten.

Sushruta Samhita: An ancient Sanskrit text on surgery and medicine believed to have been written in the 6th century BCE. It is one of the most comprehensive treatises on surgery in the world and is based on Ayurvedic principles such as doshas, Dhatus and malas.

Sushumna: One of the three main *nadis* that run along the spine.

Svadhistana: One of the seven chakras located below the navel and above the pubic bone which governs sensuality and creativity.

Tamas: One of the three *gunas* or qualities that pertain to personality and also to foods and objects. Tamas is a slow, lethargic quality.

Tikta (Bitter): One of the six tastes in Ayurveda that describes a bitter taste.

Tocopherols: A classification of organic compounds that are part of the Vitamin E family.

Triphala Powder. An herbal remedy in Ayurvedic medicine that consists of three dried fruits: amalaki, bibhitaki and haritaki. It is used to enhance digestive health and detoxification of the body.

Vata: One of the three doshas or bioenergetic constitutions in Ayurveda and is composed of air and space.

Vedanta: The end of the Vedas or sacred texts of India, with ideas coming from the Upanishads and other Vedic texts. One of the six orthodox schools of Hindu philosophy which refers to the Supreme Truth or Brahman (Universal Consciousness or Infinite Self) that underlies all reality.

Vedas: Considered among the most ancient Hindu philosophical texts in the world and are 3,000 years old. These are sacred texts that teach about ritual procedures and philosophical truths.

Vijnanamaya (Kosha): The third inner sheath of the five koshas of existence that surround the soul. It is a subtle mental sheath that consists of thinking, mind, discernment, intelligence and ego.

Vishnu Mudra: A hand position (*mudra*) used for alternate nostril breathing. It is used to gently open and close the nostrils and consists of taking one hand and wrapping your thumb over the second and third fingers, while letting the last two fingers extend as you perform the exercise. It's associated with the Hindu deity Vishnu and here the hand gesture is simply used as a yogic gesture to facilitate the breathing exercise.

Vishuddha: One of the seven chakras which is considered the throat chakra. This chakra represents communication and expansiveness.

Vitamix Blender: A high-powered blender made by the Vitamix Corporation and made from stainless steel for domestic use.

Excellent for thorough blending, juicing, pulverizing and even the blending and heating of soups.

Yoga Nidra: Yoga nidra is a deep state of relaxation in which you are still fully conscious. It is considered one of the deepest states you can attain while still fully conscious. You start by lying in corpse pose (or *savasana*) during a guided meditation that uses progressive muscle relaxation and breathing exercises in order to relax the body completely. It can also be performed in a reclining position with comfortable cushion

ABOUT THE AUTHOR

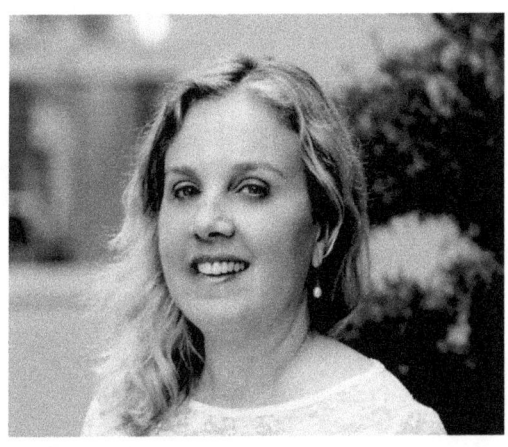

Susan Holman, MA, is a Certified Ayurvedic Consultant with a strong background in yogic science and exercise physiology. She received her MA from New York University and hosts workshops and webinars on Ayurveda and yogic science. Susan loves helping clients from all walks of life to lead their healthiest lives through Ayurveda and physical exercises. She is an animal lover and enjoys contributing to charities for animal welfare.

Susan is a keynote speaker and founder of Susan Coach LLC, a health and wellness education company. She is also an Associate Real Estate Broker in NYC. Susan is an active member of various charities and philanthropic organizations that help empower local communities. She believes everyone is entitled to optimum health and nutrition.

She is available on line and in person for Ayurvedic consultations:

Email: susan@susan.coach or book online at

http://www.wellnesschique.com

Want to learn what your dosha is in Ayurveda? Email us for details!

www.ingramcontent.com/pod-product-compliance
Lightning Source LLC
Chambersburg PA
CBHW031154020426
42333CB00013B/655